THE
HEALING
BRAIN

BREAKTHROUGH
DISCOVERIES
ABOUT HOW THE BRAIN
KEEPS US HEALTHY

Robert Ornstein
and
David Sobel

MALOR
BOOKS

This is a Malor Book
Published by ISHK
P O Box 381069, Cambridge, MA 02239-1069

First published by Simon and Schuster, 1987
This edition published by ISHK, 1999

Library of Congress Cataloging in Publication Data:
Ornstein, Robert.
    The healing brain : breakthrough discoveries about how the brain
keeps us healthy / Robert Ornstein and David Sobel.
        p.   cm.
Previously published: New York : Simon & Schuster, 1987.
Includes bibliographical references and index.
ISBN 1-883536-17-0
    1.   Medicine, Psychosomatic. 2. Brain. 3. Health. I. Sobel, David
S. (David Stuart) II. Title.
RC49.076   1999
613—dc21   98-52480
                                                       CIP

    The author is grateful for permission to use material from the
following sources:
    "Fighting Cancer: One Patient's Perspective" by N. Fiore, *New
England Journal of Medicine.*
    Neuropsychology of Human Emotion by Kenneth M. Heilman and
Paul Satz. Published by Guilford Press.
    Vulnerable, But Invincible: A Study of Resilient Children by E. E.
Werner and R. S. Smith. Published by McGraw-Hill.
    The Hardy Executive by Salvatore R. Maddi and Suzanne C. Kobasa.
Published by Dow Jones-Irwin.
    "The Faith that Heals" by Jerome D. Frank, *The Johns Hopkins
Medical Journal.*
    "Postscript" by L. D. Egbert, *Advances,* Journal of the Institute for
the Advancement of Health, 1985; 2:58.
    The Language of the Heart by James J. Lynch, Ph.D. By permission
of the author and Basic Books.

ACKNOWLEDGMENTS

We'd like to thank many of the people who helped us in the years we were working on this book: Stephen Laberge, Charles Swencionis, James Lynch. We have also had the privilege of working with almost one hundred different lecturers at our symposium, titled *The Healing Brain*. To all of you, thank you again and again for sharing your insights.

We want to thank Chris Mason for literature searches and library research. Tom Kass, Matt Budd, Christina Lepnis, Don Kemper, Meredith Minkler, and Sally Mallam all reviewed the manuscript with effort beyond that of friendship, and each has left an imprint.

THIS BOOK IS DEDICATED
TO THE SPIRIT AND TO THE INFLUENCE OF
RENÉ DUBOS.

CONTENTS

PREFACE

The brain minds the body. This idea seems so simple and central to the understanding of human health, and yet it has escaped the attention of the mainstream of medical practice and psychological thought. Medicine has largely regarded the body as a mindless machine—a perspective elucidated by a brilliant twenty-four-year-old philosopher, René Descartes, more than four hundred years ago. Proposed as a temporary expedient to permit investigation of the human organism unencumbered by the dogma of the ruling Church, this separation of mind and body has dominated medical practice and thought.

Psychology has similarly been restricted by a view that the main purpose of the human brain was to produce rational thought. Never mind that the brain is the largest organ of secretion in the body, and the neuron, far from being like a chip within a computer, is a flesh-and-blood little gland, one that produces hundreds of chemicals. These chemicals do not, for the most part, serve thought or reason. They serve keeping the body out of trouble, from commonplace problems like not falling over or walking into a wall to the myriad of tasks involved in maintaining the stability and health of the organism.

It is in the stability of our social worlds, our mental and emotional lives, and our internal physiology that health exists, and it is the brain which maintains stability by its countless adjustments, commands, and secretions.

This inconceivable organ evolved as a collection of "small brains" all living together in one body. Sometimes these brains function harmoniously, and sometimes they conflict and send mixed messages to the body. Basic to the evolution of the brain is our early attachment and dependency on other people. Our social nature links us fundamentally to others throughout our lives. When these links are strained or ruptured, the health consequences are profound.

On the positive side, the brain possesses highly refined mechanisms to maintain and restore health. We are not helpless and defenseless in the face of the stresses of everyday life. Some people seem able to view life's inevitable changes as challenges, and a study of such hardy people helps reveal why some people maintain health while others become ill.

This book is one attempt to bring about a new way of looking at the brain; not a new theory or a new study, but simply a new view. It is one which turns around the well-developed assumption that rational thought is the supreme achievement of the human brain and restores the perspective that the major role of the brain is to mind the body and maintain health.

This book, *The Healing Brain*, provides many of the raw materials for the new view: Who twenty years ago could have imagined the complex internal pain-regulation system which underlies turning off pain in response to sugar pills? Who would have thought that the death of a loved one would cause immunity to disease to plummet? Who would have thought that a sudden cardiac arrest after a shocking trauma could be due to signals deep within the brain's frontal lobe?

So the reader has to be, in the cliché, intrepid, intrepid enough to go through the varied "worlds" and disciplines of medicine, social thought, health, evolution, brain science, and psychology. We will move from beliefs to chemicals, from social interaction to high blood pressure, from grieving to suppression of immunity, so that connections—some well worked out as of now, some still yet to come—can be illuminated. Though the individual bits of evidence we present may be debated or the speculative links challenged, we believe the collective weight of the findings helps close the artificial gap between mind and body.

Rather than just presenting a series of interesting findings which link psychological states and health, we attempt, whenever possible, to highlight themes and speculate on commonalties, even, at some moments, when the research is not yet perfect. This is not, however, a final theory which ties all the observations together in one neat, simplified model, but a new perspective about what the brain is doing and about what determines health.

To begin our discussion, we take a new look at both health and the brain. Going a long way around, we start with a consideration of why the health of people in Western societies has improved over the past century. We then take a look at what the brain is actually doing.

April 1986
Robert Ornstein
David Sobel

The Stability to Resist Disease

CHAPTER ONE

IN SICKNESS AND IN HEALTH

As Roy Sampson looked down at his dying child, he was angry that the doctor had been unable to help. Sampson was a forty-five-year-old railroad worker whose child, a two-year-old girl, had become ill a week before with fever and relentless diarrhea. The doctor had visited twice before and had administered a potion that, if anything, appeared to make the sick child even worse. Sampson was all too familiar with the disease. He had already lost a child to dysentery.

It was 1887, and constant disease was common to this family. Sampson's brother had succumbed to tuberculosis, or "consumption," as it was then known. Roy remembered the uncertainty, the continuing pain, and the agony of his brother's disease. It dragged on for years and years as he watched his brother slowly waste away, consumed by coughing and fevers.

Roy and his family did everything they could think of to help, but the medical regime that was undertaken—the fasting, the purging, and the many trips to the sanitarium—did little or nothing in the end to alleviate the horror and the degeneration of his brother.

Sampson's wife had died recently, victim to a high fever that

17

followed the birth of their fifth and last child. But Roy was grateful for his own good health and because two of his own children *had* survived. Many of Sampson's friends had only one surviving child, and some had none of their children survive their first few years, even though the wife seemed almost continually in childbirth. What would these childless couples do in their old age? Who would care for them?

One hundred years later, Roy Sampson's great-great-grandson, Henry Sampson, looked down at his smiling, healthy girl. She was four, and aside from a few brief colds and an ear infection, she had been healthy all her life. Henry wasn't surprised—this was his third healthy child. The family was under good medical care. All the children made regular visits to the pediatrician. The family was protected by health insurance, and, should they become ill, a new hospital with a modern high-tech emergency room had been built only two miles away.

Disease still touched the Sampson family, but it primarily affected Henry's parents. His father had suffered his first heart attack at age fifty-four and, following his second heart attack, he underwent a complicated and expensive coronary artery bypass operation which seemed to improve his health. Henry's mother had died at age sixty after a long illness, battling uterine cancer. At the end of the treatment, his mother's doctors had tried both chemotherapy and radiotherapy, both of which failed to arrest the spread of cancer throughout her body.

These two families, generations apart, exemplify the changes in health that most people in the United States and Europe have experienced over the last century or so. In the 1800s the average life expectancy at birth was about fifty years. Today, life expectancy of a child born in the United States is well over seventy. Many people who are alive today remember vividly how the hospitals of fifty years ago were hopeless places, choked and clogged with people who suffered from incurable diseases such as tuberculosis. Then, seemingly overnight, the tuberculosis wards were emptied as this major infectious killer was almost completely knocked out by one of the first modern "wonder drugs"—streptomycin.

In the 1980s hardly a week goes by without report of a medical breakthrough: There are new developments in organ transplants;

artificial hearts; *in vitro* fertilization; drugs to lower blood-pressure and cholesterol levels; cures for impotence; instruments to peer into joints; bone-marrow transplants; new delivery systems for drugs; and inventions such as positron emission tomography and magnetic resonance imaging, which allow new ways to see into the body so that diseases can be easily diagnosed.

Many people owe their lives to the development of lifesaving antibiotics and immunizations. Smallpox is gone. Polio has nearly vanished from developed countries. Syphilis is no longer a dreaded, lethal disease. Tumors that would have killed someone defended by the medicine of 100 years ago are today removed in routine outpatient surgery. Using microsurgery, physicians can treat disorders of the eye and the knee which would have permanently disfigured or at least disabled someone only twenty-five years ago.

These important and dramatic developments have given impetus to decisions to provide ever-increasing amounts of "medical care." The United States spends more and more on medicine and its associated technology, now nearly twelve percent of the gross national product.

We don't mind spending so much, because it seems quite obvious to anyone that the developments of modern medicine are responsible for the overall dramatic improvement in health in lives like the Sampsons'.

But this assumption is wrong.

Medical treatments, especially the drug and surgical treatment of sick individuals, have had relatively little to do with the better health that people in Western societies enjoy. We are wedded to medical ideas that are incorrect.

Consider the dramatic increase in longevity that citizens of Western societies have experienced during the nineteenth and twentieth centuries. During this time the average age at death rose from about fifty to about seventy-four. But this increase in life expectancy was *not* due in the main to those medical interventions which prolonged the lives of adults.

If we look at adult lives, the changes are quite different. Roy Sampson, forty-five years old in 1887, could expect to live for about another twenty-five years. Henry Sampson at forty-five, living a century later, with all the benefit of modern medicine— the microsurgery, the image scans of the living body, the organ transplants, the beta-blockers for heart trouble, the easy availability of antibiotics, and more—could expect to live for only a few years more than his great-great grandfather, who lived before all these highly visible and dramatic developments. What lowered the death rate and increased longevity was a decline in deaths from the infectious diseases of youth. A person who survived the hazardous years of childhood was likely to live nearly as long with or without modern medicine. The rise and fall of the great epidemics of infectious diseases has more to do with social changes than medical treatments.

While plague struck Europe in the 1300s, infectious diseases like cholera, measles, smallpox, polio, and many of the respiratory viruses appear to have first become a major health problem quite late in history. These epidemics of infectious diseases began during the great social upheavals in the late Middle Ages, around the fifteenth century. These new burdens were referred to as "crowd diseases," arising with social changes which brought large concentrations of people together. At the same time, people began to make long sea expeditions in the hope that they would encounter undiscovered treasures, but often they settled for encountering undiscovered peoples—and with them, new and undiscovered diseases.

Travelers brought unfamiliar diseases to the lands they visited and carried new diseases home. There was no specific immunity to the "new germs," and "host resistance" (the ability to withstand disease) was undermined by poor nutrition and unsanitary conditions. So the germs had a field day, and unprecedented epidemics began to decimate large populations.

A French observer in the sixteenth century stated that the many diseases then plaguing his countrymen

> have scarcely anything in common except infection, such illnesses as diphtheria, *cholerine*, typhoid fever, *picotte*, smallpox, purple fever, the bosse, dendo, tac *or* harion, *the* trousse galant *or* mal chaud; *or again whooping cough*, scarlatine, *grippe*, *influenza*.

Diseases suddenly appeared and went away forever in this new mixing of germs. "Sweating sickness" ravaged England from 1486 to 1551. It affected the heart and the lungs and carried with it rheumatic pains and fits of shivering: It usually killed its hosts within a few hours. It appeared five different times and has not been seen again. Epidemics jumped from one population to another. One traveler, Alonso Montecuccoli, wrote on September

2, 1603, that he could trace the progress of the plague as it moved along the trade route. He adjusted his own business and travel plans so as to keep away from it.

But it was unavoidable: New disease traveled everywhere in the world in the sixteenth to the nineteenth centuries. Plague came into Europe from China and India via Constantinople and Egypt. Both tuberculosis and cholera arrived in the West from India in the eighteenth century.

Just as the rise of mortality from infectious diseases was occasioned by cultural and social changes, so was its decline. The decline was not due, for the most part, to medical interventions in sick individuals, but to making the environment less hazardous and improving the general resistance of people to defend themselves against germs.

These changes were the crucial part of the modern improvement in health: Deaths and disease from common infections were already declining drastically long before antibiotics, long before effective immunizations, long before effective individual medical intervention (see graphs). Look at the time course of the conquest of tuberculosis—the major cause of death in the mid-nineteenth century.

LIFE EXPECTANCY

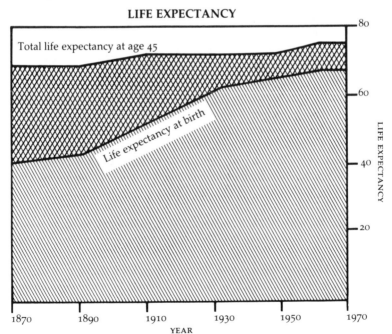

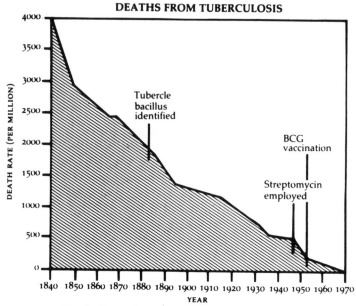

DEATHS FROM TUBERCULOSIS

Deaths from tuberculosis began to decline long before medical science provided effective treatment for it.

The death rate from tuberculosis declined from nearly three thousand deaths per million people in 1850 to fewer than twenty deaths per million today, at least as of 1973. While many drugs and severe treatments, such as surgically collapsing the lung, were tried for almost one hundred years, the first effective treatment for tuberculosis was the antibiotic streptomycin, developed in 1947. The effect of streptomycin was dramatic: Death rates from tuberculosis were quickly cut in half and declined further. Only forty years later, tuberculosis became a rarity in the West.

Most people believe the decline of tuberculosis is due to the introduction of the antibiotic. But our perspective is wrong, our time frame is wrong, and our conclusion is wrong as well. Most people are, in effect, looking only at a few exciting and vivid happenings within their lifetime, the past forty to fifty years, basing their conclusions on this familiar but very restricted evidence.

A longer view reveals that most of the total decline of deaths from tuberculosis since the 1800s occurred *before* streptomycin was first introduced. By 1945, 97 percent of the cases had already been eliminated, leaving only the remaining 3 percent to be improved by the modern medical treatments. The dramatic emptying of the hospitals that many of us and our parents have observed, then, was only the very end of the massive improvement.

Tuberculosis is not unusual: Similar reductions occurred with pneumonia, influenza, whooping cough, measles, and scarlet fever. Whooping cough (pertussis) was rampant in the late 1800s, killing over one in each thousand children. Yet today deaths from whooping cough are rare. Once again, credit often goes to the pertussis immunization, which was introduced in the 1950s. But by that time the death rate had already fallen by 90 percent

Polio is, of course, a notable exception. This viral disease was rare before the late nineteenth century, but since then has occurred in epidemics. The death rate from the disease, along with the incidence of crippling disabilities, dropped dramatically following the introduction of the polio vaccine in 1956. Nevertheless, the trend in death rates from nearly all the infectious diseases was markedly downward, with the majority of the decline occurring *before* the introduction of effective medical therapies or immunizations.

Since most of the improvement occurred before the development of specific medical interventions, what accounts for this decline of the infectious diseases? The advances in agriculture in the eighteenth and nineteenth centuries allowed people to eat much more varied and nutritious foods. Better nourished people had better immunity, too, and could thus resist better the infectious diseases. The farmer, not the doctor, was most important.

Other interventions helped: The purification of water, improved sewage disposal, and better food hygiene together account for roughly one-fifth of the total decline in infectious disease mortality. Pasteurization of milk, the food most likely to spread disease, was probably the major reason for the decrease in deaths from gastroenteritis and for the decline in infant mortality from diarrheal diseases from about 1900. Again, it was a social change, led by the food handler and sewage engineer rather than the heroics of the doctor, that deserves the credit.

Also, as more children survived the ravages of infancy and society began to provide more secure jobs, pensions, as well as social programs to care for the elderly, parents responded by choosing to have fewer babies. Had it not been for this unprecedented change in sexual behavior, long before the advent of modern methods of contraception, the population of England and Wales would have grown to 140 million rather than the 55 million it is today. The effects of such unbridled population growth on food supplies, sanitation, hygiene, and consequently on health can be imagined.

There were, of course, some medical successes, too: By the early 1900s immunizations protected against smallpox and tetanus; antitoxin treatment limited deaths from diphtheria; appendicitis and peritonitis responded to surgery; Salvarsan successfully stopped syphilis; intravenous therapy saved some with severe diarrhea; and improved obstetric care prevented childbed fever.

Today many people are alive because of the lifesaving interventions of modern medicine: the immunizations, the antibiotics, the treatment of diabetes, and the startling surgical advances including organ transplants. Many other people, while not living longer, enjoy an improved quality of life due to the advances in medical treatment for allergies, heart disease, asthma, arthritis, and pain.

Medicine has made some contribution to health, but its interventions in diseases have been greatly overemphasized as to their real effectiveness and worth to society. The contemporary health and medical effort has, in large part, been misdirected, misspent, and its successes misattributed.

The question of what improves health needs to be turned around entirely from our emphasis upon the relief of sick individuals. People are healthier today not because they receive all this well-publicized better treatment when ill, but simply because *they tend not to become ill in the first place.*

It is not as profitable as we imagine to focus almost exclusively upon "specific etiology" of diseases, spending all our research funds to isolate identifiable agents of diseases, whether they be germs, viruses, or, according to one of the terms currently in vogue, "stressors." We should rather consider the ways in which organisms remain stable in the changing world of emergencies, germs, and threats—stable to resist infection and other disorders. We might then discover the way this resistance can be strengthened.

Obviously, much of the resistance conferred is genetic: Some people, by virtue of inheriting a stronger constitution, may be able to resist disease better. Nutrition and public health measures have increased stability and thus resistance to disease, and many other measures have had this result. But there is new and much more modern evidence on this story: The evidence that the way we interact with others, the way we see ourselves as *a part of* or *apart from* other people and our society, also appears to influence general resistance to disease. These psychological and social factors are represented in brain processes, as are many of the internal systems that participate in resistance. It is the brain which is the missing link.

Not only is there new scientific evidence that connects the social world with internal states of the brain, but our medical needs themselves are now different. In many respects people in developed Western societies have reached an age of diminishing returns whereby more medical care and more and more medical expenditures will probably contribute only marginally to better health, because the increasing medical care and medical apparatus were not responsible in the first place for much of it.

Further, the benefits from the massive medical interventions must be discounted by the potential for harm. Consider the hazards of modern medicine, the so-called iatrogenic (physician-generated) diseases. These include surgical misadventures, drug reactions, missed diagnoses, and hospital-acquired infections.

One study at Boston University Medical Center found that 36 percent of patients admitted to the hospital suffered from one or more complications as a side effect of medical care. In 9 percent of patients the iatrogenic illnesses were serious, and in 2 percent contributed to the death of the patient.

Another study focused on ninety-three children who were told by their doctors that "something was wrong with their heart." When the diagnoses were evaluated it was found that only 19 percent had actual heart disease. The rest (over 80 percent) suffered only from *cardiac nondisease*, a "disorder" created entirely by misdiagnosis. The consequences of cardiac nondisease, however, are serious. Nearly half of these healthy children were restricted in their physical activity. In a subsequent study children with activity restricted as a result of their diagnosis of cardiac nondisease were found to have impaired intellectual development.

Utah and Nevada are similar in geography, climate, income, education, and degree of urbanization but are strikingly different in the health of their inhabitants. The death rate for adults is

nearly 40 percent higher in Nevada than Utah. The health differences cannot be accounted for on the basis of differences in medical care. The states have similar numbers of physicians and
hospital beds per capita.

The key differences are in the way people live. Utah is inhabited primarily by Mormons, who abstain from smoking and
drinking and have a quite rigid social organization and generally
lead quiet, stable lives. In contrast, people in Nevada prescribe
liberal doses of alcohol and tobacco for themselves and have consequently 100 to 600 percent higher death rates from cirrhosis and
lung cancer. Further, the Nevada residents are transient (more
than nine of ten Nevadans of middle age were not born in Nevada). They are "socially unstable" (in plain English this means
that Nevadans are twice as likely to be single, divorced, separated, or widowed).

There are many further indications that the way people behave,
rather than the medical care they receive, has a very great influence on their ability to resist diseases. Important evidence on this
comes from a large study of nearly seven thousand adults in
Alameda County, near San Francisco. After an initial survey
which established their health at the time, these seven thousand
people were tracked for seven years and surveyed again. Certain
health habits were identified that characterized those who remained healthy and those who became ill and died. These
"grandmother knows best" health habits included not smoking,
drinking in moderation or not at all, exercising regularly, eating
breakfast, maintaining a normal weight, eating regular meals,
and getting adequate sleep.

Consider two different forty-five-year-old men living today.
One practices five or six of these positive health habits, and the
other only one or two. The clean-living fellow can expect to live
eleven years longer than his sedentary, smoking, heavy-drinking
counterpart. Eleven years is an enormous difference considering
that the increase in life expectancy in the last century for a forty-
five-year-old man (like Roy or Henry Sampson) was considerably
less. And this gain—which took the century of immense effort,
massive funding, research developments, testing, and retesting
that has gone into modern scientific medicine—is less than the
difference a person potentially has in his or her own control.

It is a shameful waste of billions of dollars and millions of lives.
Why should we place our faith and resources in a medicine based

largely on the treatment of diseases? Why spend 12 percent of our gross national product on medical care? Why is the largest single budget expense in a new General Motors automobile not the steel, not the design work, not the factory expenses, but the cost of health insurance for the workers involved? We should be studying what really controls our bodies and our health.

Health itself is difficult to see and to quantify. Preventing disease is a peculiar business in which one must gain satisfaction more from what does *not* happen that from what does. The absence of an automobile accident, the protection from an infectious disease, or the unseen prevention of a possible suicide attracts less attention (and funding) than the heroics of a trauma surgeon, the cure with antibiotics, or the pharmacological reversal of a drug overdose.

It is understandable that we know very little about health, since there is always a strong need to respond to and care for those who are sick. It is far simpler, much easier, more exciting, and more personally satisfying to look for the dramatic medical "magic bullets," for dramatic surgical rescues, than it is to weigh, judge, and confirm the more complex determinants of health like behavior, estranged social relationships, and deleterious environments.

Medical scientists are just beginning to break free of their early and simplistic engineering mentality. This oversimplified approach, a way of doing science always useful at the beginning, attempted to understand all relevant aspects of health in physical and chemical terms. Medical scientists looked only to biology and analyzed the structure and mechanical functioning of the human body in fine detail.

Anatomy, physiology, biochemistry, and molecular biology were considered the "basic medical sciences," and psychiatry, with its emphasis upon mental causes of diseases, was in another department (probably in another building); social and emotional factors were not even on the chart. "Real" diseases were definable organic diseases. Medical therapy consisted of physical and chemical interventions in the "body machine," the way a garage mechanic would do a valve job on the family car. Disease was essentially a technical problem requiring a technical solution.

Yet the word *health* appears everywhere: "*health* care system," *"health* care providers," *"health* science expenditures," *"health* maintenance organizations." Some medical schools are now called "health science centers." With all the discussion of "health care," one might have imagined there would have been some understanding of it.

Nearly all the talk of "health" is about the care for the sick— we have what might be better called a "disease care system." And the relationship between disease or sickness care and health is tenuous at best.

Providing more and more medical care does not necessarily produce healthier people; a healthy population is one that does not get sick in the first place, rather than one that gets sick and then is returned to health by medical care. There is more to be gained by a thorough study of how organisms avoid illness than there is from the study of disease agents alone.

The most brilliant, successful, and influential approach to the study of disease agents was Louis Pasteur's germ theory of disease. Yet even in his early studies of the diseases of silkworms, as Pasteur elaborated this central discovery of modern medicine, he was aware of the alternative: that host resistance could be strengthened.

In the 1870s the silk industry in France was nearly wiped out by a disease that attacked the developing silkworm. Pasteur was called upon to stop the disease, which he discovered was caused by a protozoan. He demonstrated that the disease could be controlled by eliminating the microbe from the silkworm nurseries.

However, Pasteur also noticed that it was not just the presence of the germ but the physiological state of the silkworm that also determined the susceptibility to infection. While his later studies with anthrax and rabies still reflected his focus on the agents of disease, he later noted: "If I were to undertake new studies on the silkworm disease, I would concern myself with the ways of increasing their general vigor . . . I am convinced that it would be possible to discover techniques for giving worms a higher level of robustness and thereby rendering them more resistant to infection."

In addition to his interest in the causative role of microorganisms in disease, he was also aware of the importance of what he called the *"terrain"*—the environmental factors which determined susceptibility and resistance to disease. In fact, Pasteur and his colleague and contemporary Claude Bernard long debated whether the disease producer, the microbe, or the body's equilibrium were more important. Pasteur sometimes reflected that "the road not taken" might have been more profitable and that the body's biochemical and physiological state, even emotional states, profoundly affects the course and outcome of infectious disease.

He was so concerned with this point that on his deathbed he said, *"Bernard avait raison. Le germe n'est rien, c'est le terrain qui est tout"* (Bernard was right. The germ is nothing, the soil is everything). While Pasteur may have gone a little too far in his assessment of his work at the moment of his death—certainly the germ is not "nothing"—he may have been reacting to the out-of-balance and simplistic medicine he helped to create.

While some infectious agents, such as measles, cause symptoms in nearly everyone exposed, this is the exception rather than the rule. In most cases exposure to an infectious agent is not sufficient to cause disease. Why does one person who is exposed become ill, while another remains symptom-free? The difference lies in the "resistance of the host." Previous exposure to the infectious agent either naturally or through immunization can stimulate immunity. Immunity also can be influenced by genetic constitution and nutritional factors. But now there is evidence that brain processes can influence immunity to infectious diseases.

Consider tuberculosis. Presence of the tubercle bacillus is necessary but not sufficient to explain the onset or course of the disease; many people who are exposed to this pathogenic agent do not become infected. And of those infected, only 5 to 15 percent become clinically ill. As early as 1919 researchers studying tuberculosis observed a decrease in the activity of white blood cells in patients during emotional excitement. Many had severe life crises in the one to two years preceding the onset or relapse of the disease.

It was even then hypothesized that the "stress of contemporary life" could impair immunological function, thus increasing susceptibility to tuberculosis. But these observations were not followed up until the 1970s when technical advances made brain-immune connections feasible to study scientifically.

At the time, there was great hope that cures such as those found for syphilis would be found for everything. So the "magic bullet" approach to disease has ignored psychological and social factors in the development, course, and resolution of diseases. The focus on pathology of most medical scientists (we almost wrote "pathological focus") has made scant the development of knowledge of how to bolster the body and how to strengthen the resistance to disease. Ironically, scientists in agriculture and animal husbandry have given more effort to producing environmental and nutritional milieus that foster disease resistance. In this sense, our livestock have better health care than we do.

With the reduction in mortality from acute infectious disease in most parts of the developed world, the kinds of illnesses we now suffer are different: As tuberculosis replaced sweating sickness and other diseases, now chronic degenerative diseases like heart disease, stroke, cancer, arthritis, cirrhosis, chronic lung disease, and mental illness predominate. These multifactorial diseases are not suitable to the methods of trying to isolate a single cause. As Henry Dixon points out, "The dazzling achievements of specific etiology have now been followed by a situation where all of our major health problems—most obviously cardiovascular disease, cancers, and much mental illness—represent areas where the theory has failed." We need to consider multiple causes and re-open consideration of psychological and social forces as determinants of disease.

This book is an attempt to look ahead, to look beyond the evidence we now possess, an attempt to redirect our ideas of what the brain is for, and how we might improve health. As with any such attempt, there are holes and gaps in the current evidence, but the overall shape of the argument is, we think, becoming clear. It is our belief that there is a new understanding arising in the health, psychological, and brain sciences: To understand health is to understand the central role of the brain in maintaining the resistance of the body.

The general disregard of social and mental factors in health mirrors the attitude in the 1800s when surgeons ridiculed the concept of antisepsis and the germ theory of disease. The surgeons persisted in operating in unclean surroundings, sometimes defiantly sharpening their scalpels on the soles of their shoes to show their contempt for the putative power of invisible germs. Similarly, the current ignorance and insensitivity to the "invisible" symbolic messages in human interactions, including those between doctor and patient, limits the effectiveness of contemporary medicine.

In some ways the shift from an emphasis on sickness to an

emphasis on health has just begun, although the initial under-standing is oversimplified. In popular medical columns, in pop-ular magazines, the message is disseminated that something called "life-style" is the culprit. The "new germs" of today are bad habits such as smoking, risk factors such as broad changes in "life events," and the extreme psychological reactions to environ-mental disruptions such as job loss or divorce. These are now viewed as the modern external agents that attack us and produce modern "disorders" like "stress."

Yet even these "bad actions" and potential stressors are not sufficient to explain who gets sick and who stays healthy. Heart disease is the leading cause of death and sickness in the devel-oped countries. Through years of research several key "risk fac-tors" have been discovered. These factors (which may be behavioral or biological) increase the probability of developing coronary heart disease: Cigarette smoking, elevated serum cho-lesterol, and elevated blood pressure are the most important. The evidence seems strong and compelling. People who have one of these risk factors have twice the likelihood of developing coro-nary heart disease; those with two factors are 3.5 times as likely, and those with all three risk factors have nearly 6.0 times greater probability of developing heart disease.

But the obvious conclusion is misleading: *Knowing whether a person smokes, has high blood pressure, or elevated cholesterol does very little to predict who will have a heart attack.* A comprehensive look at the evidence suggests something different. Combining the data from the six major heart disease projects shows that of the sev-enty-three hundred men in the studies, six hundred had high values for all three of the risk factors. Yet of this group of six hundred high-risk men, only eighty-two suffered a heart attack during the ten years of follow-up study. So *86 percent of those who had the very highest risk for heart attacks did not have a heart attack over the ten years of study.*

Further, of the twenty-two hundred men with two of the risk factors, 91 percent suffered no heart attack. Conversely, the vast majority of people who *did* have a heart attack did not have all of the major risk factors. This is not to suggest that smoking, ele-vated cholesterol, or high blood pressure are not important, but only that they do surprisingly little to predict who stays healthy and who becomes ill. Attention is again misdirected to a few dramatic factors, as it was in the consideration of tuberculosis.

So it is not only germs that attack and that can be killed by a "magic bullet," and it is not only those horrible lurking stressors and risk factors that kill. We and medicine should turn around the questions of health and disease and focus not upon those few fortunate people who are relieved of their illnesses by medical means, but to consider those, far greater in numbers, who do not become ill or who in the face of disease move towards health.

It is important to get away from an idea that one is either sick or not, healthy or not, and to look instead at the person as a balancing act of these forces, sometimes stable, sometimes not; sometimes not sick, but with perhaps 20 percent of a flu, sometimes with a full outbreak, sometimes with pain, sometimes not. The person changes, grows up, grows old, is in contact with more or fewer germs, is happy or depressed, is married or divorced, enraged or calm. And the germs evolve as well.

The maintenance of health is a remarkable balancing act. In this book we will try to look at the center of this balancing act, the brain, and consider why seemingly unrelated factors like the strength of one's social relationships increase the strength of one's resistance to disease. This is not a new approach: "It is much more important to know what sort of patient has the disease than what sort of disease the patient has," wrote Sir William Osler around the turn of the century. But it is an approach for which there is now a new convergence of evidence: from studies on the role of medicine; from research on brain chemistry; from the discovery of missing links between the immune and cardio-vascular systems and mental states; from an understanding that the brain is more like a collection of messy and wet glands than it is like a cool computer; and from a renewed appreciation that the human organism is not a mindless machine.

The Brain Minds the Body

BODYGUARDS

Why does your blood pressure drop when you touch your pet?

Why should hostility bring about heart attacks, and why doesn't anger?

Why do widowers die at a rate three times greater than other men of comparable age?

Why do people who lose their jobs have increased rates of heart disease and lung disorders, no matter what their occupation?

Changes in the social world. Changes in emotional and mental states. At first glance, it may seem that these changes have little to do with disease. But "real," organic diseases are linked to changed beliefs about oneself, to the nature of one's relationship to others, and one's position in the social world.

Such links only appear impossible, or at least irrelevant or unimportant, from the early and simplistic medical view, which regards the body as a mindless automaton. Our hearts, lungs, stomach, immune systems, and all other organs are hardly independent, autonomous organs. Certainly they have autonomous functions, but they are regulated by and in communication with the brain.

Many different factors, from molecules to mitochondria, from cells to the self, from spouses to societies, can affect health. There may be specific disturbances in the organs of the body, an inborn error in the genes, a break in personal relationships, a radical change in one's job prospects, a shift in the government, or an improvement in economic conditions; all of these can occur separately and independently, yet each one can destabilize the organism and contribute to the onset or to the progress of disease.

Disease and disorders have multiple causes and can occur for many different reasons, so any disease, mental or physical, is rarely all "in the mind" of those afflicted, nor is it an inevitable consequence of the attack of "germs" on the body. There is no simple equation; rather we should view health as a constant battle between the strength of the attack and the stability of the defense. The patient is neither always responsible for the disease nor always helpless. Some disorders overwhelm anyone's good intentions and clean living, and sometimes seeming irrelevancies such as watching a movie can affect the immune system. It is not simple. Many factors, from the state of one's marriage to the current state of hormone production, are managed instant by instant by one three-pound lump of tissue containing 100 billion, give or take a few billion, cells.

The answers about the relationship of the brain, mind, health, and society are hardly all in, but the evidence from many different areas of research now available begins to make some of the connections clear. The heart itself cannot decide that loss of a loved one is too much for it; the liver alone does not see the shame of embarrassment; the immune system does not know whether its client is employed or not, divorced or not.

The brain does.

The brain minds the body: the function of the internal organs, the safety and stability of the individual, and the social body of human society. Health maintenance is the *primary* function of the brain, not rational thought, language, poetry, and other functions usually thought of as "the brain." The brain has evolved complex "bodyguards," designed to protect and maintain health.

A rather haphazard and seemingly disorganized set of structures makes up the brain, because the brain was built, partly by "design," partly by accident, by the processes of evolution over hundreds of millions of years. Think of it as a crazily built old house, "ramshackle" as Robert Ornstein, Dick Thompson, and David Macaulay described it in *The Amazing Brain*, like a house that was originally built long ago for a small family, then added on to, over several generations of growth and changes.

So it is with the original structure of the brain, the "old rooms." The brain contains "room" after "room" of different structures united because they are in the same skull, side by side. The human brain is not like a well-designed modern house, one in which each cubic foot is well planned and organized. We were just not built that way. We carry our evolution inside us, within the different structures of the brain, structures built in different eras. There are many different little brains inside the skull.

There is an archaeology as well as an architecture to the brain, as it was built up over millions of years. As with an archaeological dig, there are "layers" to the brain. The human brain was not constructed of new elements. It is a compendium of circuits piled atop one another, most of the circuits developed to serve a short-term purpose in millennia past. Evolution does not work for the long term, but for the immediate exigencies of survival for individuals. Brain structures which evolved to aid adaptation of earlier species may be co-opted, remodeled, and put to different use in the human brain.

The brain evolved, as is well known by now, in different levels, each one designed to maintain stability in its organism as animals moved from the sea, to land, to the trees, to the savannahs of East Africa, to Fifth Avenue. The early layers and the "higher" brain structures share the same head, the same neurons, and the same blood supply. The neurochemicals which are activated for emergencies may course through the entire structure. An instability in one brain system can easily come to affect others, as a fire started in one dwelling of a large apartment building affects the neighbors, even though they did not cause the fire.

The oldest and deepest area of the brain evolved more than 500 million years ago, before the evolution of mammals. Many scientists refer to this part as the "reptilian brain," since the human brain stem looks like that of a reptile. The brain stem is primarily concerned with the fundamental biological stability of the organism and manages the first and the simplest means of life support —such as the control of breathing and heart rate, and general warnings about the approach of possible predators or prey. These brain systems were sufficient for the ocean life of our ancestors.

From about 300 to 200 million years ago, during the transition from sea-dwelling animals to those which lived on land, a new brain had to evolve. "Living off the land" causes many problems for the brain. Life in the sea is relatively stable and easy compared to the changing environment on land. There is no harsh winter, or at least there is extremely little temperature variation, so there is no need for the organism to regulate internal temperature. Gravity is less of a problem in the buoyant ocean environment. One does not have to worry much about where one's next drink is coming from, so complicated systems for thirst regulation and fluid retention are hardly worth evolving.

But to maintain the stability of the body on land with its vagaries—the irregular supplies of food and drink, the extremes of climate and new dangers unknown in the deep—a new and different brain grew. This area of the brain was named the limbic system, a group of cell structures in the center, sitting immediately atop the brain stem.

It is often called the "mammalian brain," because the same brain structure is found in all land mammals. The limbic system is the area of the brain that helps to maintain "homeostasis," a stable environment within the body. Homeostatic mechanisms located in the limbic system regulate such functions as the maintenance of body temperature, blood pressure, heart rate, and blood sugar level.

But it does much more than just control recurrent internal processes: In land mammals the limbic system increases control and is involved in the elaborate emotional reactions that have to do with survival, such as self-protection through fighting or escaping. It contains the *hypothalamus*—the "brain of the brain," its most intricate and amazing structure. It regulates eating, drinking, sleeping, waking, body temperature, hormone balances, heart rate, sex, and emotions.

When the hypothalamus is injured, the animal may not eat or drink, no matter how long it has been deprived of food or water. Conversely, stimulation or destruction of certain areas of the hypothalamus causes incessant eating, which can be fatal.

The hypothalamus operates through feedback. Body temperature is registered in specialized neurons in the hypothalamus which respond to the temperature of incoming blood as it circulates through the brain. If the blood is too cool, the hypothalamus stimulates heat production and conservation.

Through a combination of electrical and chemical messages, the hypothalamus directs the master gland of the brain, the pituitary. This gland regulates the body through hormones (chemicals manufactured and secreted by special neurons in the brain), which are carried through the blood to specific "target cells" in the body. The pituitary synthesizes most of the hormones used by the brain to communicate with the major glands of the body.

The latest level of the brain to develop, the cerebral cortex, made its appearance in modern form about 50 million years ago.

It performs the functions that increase adaptability and is responsible for the characteristics which make us most human. In the cortex decisions are made; the external and internal world is organized; individual experiences are stored in memory; speech is produced and understood; paintings are seen; music is heard.

The cortex is a thin, enfolded layer only about one-eighth of an inch thick. If it were spread out, it would be about the size of a newspaper page. Of all mammals, human beings have the most enfolded cortex, perhaps because such a large cortex had to fit into a small head to permit passage through a narrow birth canal.

The cortex is built in a quite interesting manner, with specialized cells arranged in columns, columns which seem to have specific functions. For example, certain columns of cells in the visual cortex are specialized to detect corners or edges of objects in the visual field. These standard ("hard-wired") data-processing centers in the cortex and brain structures below serve as "modules" for the basic processing and interpretation of information. So the "rooms" of the brain have their own columns!

Inside the cortex lie separate centers with specific functions, which we like to call talents. Mathematical ability is a separate talent from the ability to move gracefully; verbal agility is distinct from the previous two. There is a range of different functions, for smelling, for thinking, for moving, for calculating that the brain possesses, and they are not all given equally to each of us; people are not as consistent as we might have imagined. If you look at the brain this way, you will see that it is not a single organ but divided into different and well-defined areas, each of which possesses a rich concentration of certain abilities.

The cortex is responsible for making decisions and judgments on all the information coming into it from the body and the outside world. It first receives information from the outside world; analyzes and compares it with stored information of prior experiences and knowledge, and makes a decision; then sends its own messages and instructions out to the appropriate muscles, glands, and other organs. The cortex is the "seat" of the rational abilities we develop.

But the brain, as a whole, and as this tour of five hundred thousand millennia in a few paragraphs might begin to indicate, is *not* primarily designed for thinking. Those attributes we consider most human—language, perception, and intelligence—represent only a *small fraction of the brain's functions.* The academic and scientific analysis of the brain has been focused wrongly on these, admittedly interesting, functions of the brain.

In brain and cognitive science much of the research effort is on those attributes which are most uniquely human: language, thought, creativity, intelligence, and logic. Our models of the brain compare it to an information-processing machine; now the computer, years ago the switchboard. Brain scientists have confused our own ideal of what we would like to be—rational decision makers—with our analysis of what the brain is actually doing. Thought came very late in the day of the brain, intelligence came later, at least as we understand it, and it is a real question whether rationality has come at all.

The brain's primary responsibility is to help the organism avoid trouble. From this point of view it would be quite surprising if the brain did not have some influence on control of the functioning of all body systems. The immune system, the diffuse system of cells which guard our bodies from foreign invaders, was once thought to be immune to nervous system control and mental influence. This viewpoint was more a sign of the immaturity of medical science, which found it difficult to understand the complexity of the immune system, let alone relate it to the soft (read "unscientific") world of the mind.

Thinking that different systems of the body act autonomously (there was even the idea of an "autonomic nervous system") took hold in the era when both neurophysiology and medicine were at their beginnings. The magic bullet successes of mechanistic interventions into diseased bodies made those who were interested in the effects of the brain on health somewhat suspect.

The one discipline which considered these factors—psychiatry —was placed in another department from the "hard sciences" like immunology and biochemistry. No matter the academic mistakes; it is all one organism with all organ systems under some degree of control by brain mechanisms. Asking whether the brain "knows" about the immune system is like asking whether President Richard Nixon knew about Watergate.

The link between the brain and the other internal organs is not to be "made" anew by us in this book: It is there (and always was), because the brain is another organ of the body. It grows as a part of and develops along with the rest of the body with built-in connections to the other organs. It does not grow up in the midst of silicon chips or disk drives to be inserted into the skull later on.

The brain has a body to manage. It controls temperature, blood flow, and digestion; it monitors every sensation, breath and heartbeat, every blink and swallow. It directs movement: Walk this way, take the hand off the hot stove, lift the arm to catch the ball, smile. The tongue, the lungs, the mouth, and the pharynx all must be directed to move to produce speech. All these actions are not designed primarily for poetry or opera, but for communication, to preserve the safety, stability, and health of the body which owns the brain.

If we followed this line of thought about the brain, our ideas and research efforts would undergo an important change; and we could turn around concepts of health and disease.

Its real job is involved enough: In order to function in a complex environment, actions must be planned, guided, and organized: We must know when and where to walk; when to speak and what to say; when to eat, drink, eliminate, and sleep. These actions must be coordinated with events in the outside world.

The brain responds to changes in the external and internal worlds. Through the senses the brain receives information about occurrences in the outside world. The internal state of the body, such as blood sugar level and body temperature, are controlled, in part, by the central nervous system. The stimulus that gets the brain's attention is one that signals a change from the existing state. The change may be as subtle as a change in air pressure or as jarring as a novel or unexpected statement. The brain constantly interprets information it receives, "matching" it against a "model" it develops of the world.

The brain is the major organ of adaptation. It tells the body what to do based on its information on the changing state of the world. The ability to respond quickly to change and to be flexible in responding are the primary ingredients of adaptability, both physical and psychological. The more complex the organism, the more options for flexibility and adaptation. Consider what happens when a frog is confronted by a fallen tree. The frog has such a specialized sensory system and brain that it probably will not notice the tree unless it runs into it; it does not "see" the tree as we do. A human can cut it, play seesaw on it, make tables out of it, or even make paper for this book. This greater flexibility of action that characterizes the human adaptation is in large part due to a larger and more complex brain.

As we evolved upon the biological underpinnings of fishes, rats, and monkeys, which were developed and elaborated in early homonids, it should not be surprising that we have many different kinds of needs, many ways of satisfying them, and that we are doing thousands of things at any moment. In dealing with this continuous flux of input and output, the brain must have evolved some sort of way of simplifying this complexity, a priority system to signal what is important to deal with and what can be safely ignored or temporarily put on the back burner. It is, somehow, the brain's job to keep track of this system of continuously shifting priorities.

Thus there is an innate priority system in the brain: Certain events seem to enter our consciousness much more easily than others. Suppose you are having a discussion about your marriage. It may seem quite important at the moment, but what happens when you get a cinder in your eye or put your hand on a flame? Even the most compelling argument disappears! Pain can flood consciousness in the same way that a crisis fills the front page of a newspaper. The priority system gives certain events, those affecting survival, fast access inside. Survival and safety come first—while hunger will not intrude as dramatically as pain does, the need for food will be felt if left unattended.

It is useful to picture all these different kinds of requirements forming a "pyramid," as did psychologist Abraham Maslow. At the bottom are the most basic needs; as one progresses to the top, the needs and the goals become more complex. The relative strength of the different needs, called "prepotence," distinguishes the levels of the hierarchy. The "stronger" needs are lower: Given the lack of both friendship and water, the need for water is stronger, "prepotent." It will preempt consciousness until it is satisfied.

The brain shifts up and down a constantly changing set of priorities, keeping balance, keeping the cells of the body properly hydrated and with a mineral content close to that of the sea, organizing Sunday afternoon parties with the family, adjusting heart rate in response to a stressor, alerting the body when a loud noise is heard, planning the next slide show presentation, shunting blood around the body, maintaining weight, and thousands more, wheeling and healing along.

The many different and separate systems within the brain, cohabiting in the same skull, are there for the purpose of surviving biologically, for which health is the primary prerequisite. An organism that is sick is unlikely to reproduce. An organism that has accidents does not survive to produce many offspring. Remember, many organisms lived for quite a while before human beings came upon the scene, and those that remain have had to do something correctly in order to keep healthy for the last 500 million years.

Technical note: This period begins 499,999,960 years before the effective administration of streptomycin, and 499,999,925 years before Salvarsan.

So, a long time ago, when the world was very different, when Georgia almost touched Ghana—before the present physical and created world—our ancestors had already evolved many different highly effective and interdependent programs, which resided within different brain structures, to keep their bodies stable and healthy in the face of internal and external demands and disruptions. Some of these bodyguards remain effective in modern conditions, like the exquisite control of the oxygenation of the blood or the temperature of the body under widely different conditions, and the precise regulation of weight.

These intrinsic healing and self-regulatory systems of the brain may at first glance seem dull and commonplace, but they should not be overlooked in favor of the striking medical successes: They are vital to our health. Many are so common and obvious that they attract little notice, personally or scientifically. Yet it is often the malfunction or breakdown of these brain-managed bodyguards that makes the organism vulnerable to disease in the first place and necessitates medical intervention.

Why do people cry? Recent evidence suggests that the tears produced by emotional crying may be a way that the body disposes of toxic substances. It may seem strange to think of crying as beneficial. Yet many people say that "a good cry" makes them feel better.

The belief that crying has positive effects is of ancient origin. More than two thousand years ago, Aristotle theorized that crying at a drama "cleanses the mind" of suppressed emotions by a process called catharsis—the reduction of distress by releasing the emotions. Many people attend movies and plays that they know beforehand are, shall we say, "elicitors of psychogenic lacrimation," or tearjerkers. Such people may cry freely in movies and may delight in the experience.

There have been a few studies of the health effects of crying. Borquist in 1906 obtained reports of the effects of crying, including the observation of fifty-four of fifty-seven respondents that crying had positive results. Herbert Weiner found from reports that asthma attacks—long thought to be largely psychosomatic—may cease as a result of crying.

While the research on the benefits of crying is intriguing but hardly decisive, other strands of evidence are becoming available. Tears produced by emotional crying such as those elicited by those tearjerker movies differ in chemical content from those caused by irritants such as onion juice. Emotional tears contain more protein than tears induced by irritants. William Frey contends that emotional crying is an eliminative process in which tears actually remove toxic substances from the body.

Crying may "cleanse the mind" in a much more literal sense than even the catharsis theorists imagine. Other researchers are now examining the contents of emotional tears for substances such as endorphins, ACTH, prolactin, and growth hormone, all of which are released by stress. While the research on psychoactive substances in tears is just beginning, there is reason to think that emotional tears may be important in the maintenance of physical health and emotional balance.

Why do we develop a fever with an infection? The elevated temperature may be part of a brain-initiated reaction to help fight infections. When the body is infected, chemicals called pyrogens are released into the bloodstream. Pyrogens act on temperature-sensing neurons in the hypothalamus to reset the thermostat to a higher temperature. And setting the temperature higher seems to be effective. Experiments in which animals are prevented from raising their body temperature in response to an infection have higher death rates, suggesting that the fever fights the infection.

How this occurs is not known for certain. One theory holds that at higher body temperatures iron is less available in the bloodstream and the replication of germs, which requires iron, is impeded. Current medical thinking has shifted from reducing the fever with drugs such as aspirin (unless the fever is extremely high or the person is debilitated) to appreciating the role of this brain-controlled reaction.

Pain, too, is information of great priority to the organism and is a special experience to the person. It is so important that it is organized as a separate system within the central nervous system. Pain information travels through circuitry that seems carefully designed: from quite special receptors into a special network of priority systems in transmission to the brain. Pain is one way we keep out of trouble.

Similarly, sneezes, shivers, and many other innate reactions have their own specific health functions. These are all controlled by brain mechanisms, responding to the need to keep the organism stable.

These common reactions are not accidents and are not trivial compared with the rationality of our elaborate medical care system. They are important parts of the brain's management of the body; they guard us from diseases and disorders, maintain body weight and temperature, fight infections, avoid poisons, keep things stable, and maintain health.

These "health maintenance programs" evolved in our predecessors long before the higher levels of the brain developed. They are reliable systems since they are below conscious control and are not affected by conscious decisions of the organism. Have you ever gone to a restaurant and found the food spoiled, so much that you have been unable to return, even though you have had many good experiences there and would like to go back? In this case you can almost feel the operation of the health maintenance system taking over, making sure you are disgusted at the thought of going back and overriding any bright ideas or rational thoughts you might have. Why does it work that way?

It is generally considered a "good thing" across all cultures (and across all species as far as we know) not to get poisoned. Few species with an appetite for truly poisonous dishes would survive long enough to contribute their genes to the pool of ancestors. We, too, seem to have many built-in guards against such poisonings, and in us the effects can color preferences for travel, for aesthetics, and more commonly, for our taste (and smell), since taste is intimately related to detecting nutritious versus poisonous things.

One of those experiences happened to one of the authors, Robert Ornstein, who relates:

> I don't eat Mexican food. My friends always make fun of me because of this. You're so inconsistent, they tell me; you love hot food, like

Indian curry; you love tomatoes, onions, garlic, avocados. It seems strange to me too; it's not just that I don't care for the food, I simply *can't bear* the thought of eating it, no matter what, no matter how hungry I am. It seems quite odd.

I know when and where I developed my problem. About twenty-five years ago I was working as a deckhand on a freighter that stopped at the port of Zihuatanejo, on the west coast of Mexico. We arrived one night and I went ashore to enjoy a meal given for the ship's crew. The ship left "Z" early the next morning.

It was my time to stand watch on the bow. Before the sun came up a violent storm arose. The rain poured, the wind blew, and the bow of the ship leaped time and again out of the water, crashing again and again into the sea. Again and again the ship heaved. The only way I could stand up to stand watch out there was to tie myself onto the little perch on the bow. So I bounced and heaved (in more than one sense of the word!) along with the ship itself.

When all had calmed down, I returned to my quarters, sick and completely exhausted. I slept for twelve hours. When I awoke I was afraid of returning to the bow of the ship, and I was completely disgusted by the idea of Mexican food. My fear of the bow was, I think, completely understandable, but I got over that fast. I returned to my regular watch two or three days later. However, I have never been able to eat Mexican food again, even though I "knew" the cause of my sickness was the storm, not the dinner, so deeply into the mind went the association of the dinner with the sickness.

There is a body of literature on how the brain is wired up to learn about certain health-related experiences. Martin Seligman proposed that there is a continuum of biological "preparedness" for different experiences. John Garcia has shown, in conditioning studies, that rats are "prepared" to associate nausea with taste but not with other external events. Doesn't this make sense? How well would a rat survive if it decided it was sick because of something it heard or saw? Or a rat that reacted to a sore foot with "it must be something I ate"?

That's why I have, for all these years, been unable to eat Mexican food. Of the particular combination of events I experienced, only the meal and the stomach upset—not the storm and the tossing ship—became strongly associated, because the ability to quickly learn the relationship between specific food and stomach upset is strongly built in to us. My association is specific, just for Mexican food—not for Mexican clothing, furniture, art, the Mayan ruins, and the like.

I behaved like a subject in one of these rat torture experiments. Even now that I know *why* I can't eat Mexican food, I still can't do anything about it—my "prepared associations" are stronger than I am. I have had to play tricks on myself, not all of which are successful. I have convinced myself that guacamole is really California food and that chili and nachos are from Texas. And the brain does not only deter us from eating poisons once experienced; it governs the metabolism of all the food we eat as part of its health maintenance.

Internal stability operates by feedback routines, like those of a thermostat. If the set point of a thermostat is 68 degrees Fahrenheit, external temperatures much higher than that cause the cooling systems to come on, whereas temperatures below 68 degrees result in heat production. Other processes work the same way. We eat when we are hungry; we are hungry when our body needs more fuel. When cold we shiver, which warms us up. Sweat cools us off when we are hot.

Temperature regulation works via the same feedback principles as a thermostat. The set point temperature, usually 98.6°F (37°C) is maintained by a system of *thermometer neurons* located in the hypothalamus. They measure blood temperature: If there is a discrepancy of about 1°C from the set point, they alter their firing rate, which triggers actions either to warm or cool the blood. Warming is accomplished by increasing muscle tone and shivering, which increases heat production, and by curling up and constricting blood vessels in the skin to diminish heat loss. Cooling is achieved by loss of fluid through sweating and vasodilation in the arms, legs, and head.

Fluids, to us land animals, are essential: Every cell of the body is bathed in them, they have a mineral concentration similar to the sea, and they constitute 75 percent of body weight. The maintenance of proper fluid intake and regulation is an extremely important and intricate job, since a small loss of fluid or change in concentration of the electrolytes in the body fluids can kill us.

When your mouth feels dry, you drink—it seems so simple. However, there is a complicated brain-directed system which regulates body fluids. Your mouth is dry because there is a drop in the water content of the blood; this dries out the salivary glands. Usually the glands dry out gradually, but this drying may occur suddenly, as when the body exercises on a hot day.

However, thirst can be quenched in several ways, only one of which is wetting the salivary glands. Water placed directly into the stomach through a tube reduces thirst. There is a more central mechanism for fluid control than the glands in the mouth. When the water content outside the cells (primarily in the blood) drops, the concentration of salt (which is usually 0.9 percent) in bodily fluids increases. That causes fluid from the cells to be released into the bloodstream, increasing blood volume and hence blood pressure.

Pressure receptors in blood vessels also detect even the smallest reduction in the water content of the blood. This leads, by means of messages transmitted from the vessels by the sympathetic nervous system, to the release of renin, an enzyme produced by the kidney. Renin changes blood protein into a new compound, a "thirst substance," which acts on receptors in the hypothalamus and other parts of the limbic system. This activates the sensation of thirst.

How we know to stop drinking is less clear than why we start, because we stop before the fluid has time to enter the cells of the body. Pressure receptors in the blood vessels detect entering fluid, then they reduce renin production, which diminishes the activity in the area of the hypothalamus concerned with thirst. This cannot be the whole story, because much of the liquid is still unabsorbed when we cease drinking—perhaps increased stomach volume is used as a feedback signal as well.

If there is no fluid intake, as occurs in sleep, and fluids within cells are too low, a hormonal feedback system is activated. The anterior hypothalamus produces antidiuretic hormone (ADH), which signals the kidneys to divert some of the water in the urine to the bloodstream. The absence of ADH, which may result from damage to the hypothalamus, as in the disease *diabetes insipidus*, leads to an increase of ten to fifteen times the normal amount of urine and almost constant thirst and drinking.

Thirst regulation is more complex than temperature regulation, and the processes regulating hunger are even more complex than those regulating thirst. While disorders of temperature regulation and thirst are unusual, hunger disorders such as obesity are common.

It seems obvious that we know when we are hungry, but as with thirst there is a complex system underlying our experience. *Gastric* and *metabolic* factors tell us when to eat and when to stop.

Walter Cannon cajoled his research assistant into swallowing a balloon attached to a graph that recorded the changes in size of the balloon. When the stomach expanded or contracted, so did the balloon. Cannon's assistant's reports of hunger pangs coincided with contractions of the balloon. Cannon proposed that stomach contractions were the primary signal of hunger.

There is more to hunger than stomach contractions and more to stomach contractions than stomach emptiness. Stomach contractions stop when sugar is injected into the bloodstream, even though the stomach is empty. Metabolic factors relate hunger to the maintenance of energy and body weight. They are registered in the brain in terms of level of blood sugar and the amount of fat deposited in the body.

We get hungry when our blood sugar (glucose) is low, but we do not stop eating only because blood sugar is restored to the proper level. The control of eating is complex. It is mediated by several brain structures including the hypothalamus. When the lateral hypothalamus (LH) of a rat is destroyed, the rat will stop eating and will starve to death without tube feeding.

Destruction of the ventromedial nuclei (VMN) of the hypothalamus results in hyperphagia or extreme overeating. This produces fat rats who are unable to stop eating. These rats are picky eaters who consume an enormous amount, but they only eat a lot of what they like—the same with obese human beings. Obese human beings and rats with VMN lesions have lost sensitivity to internal cues like stomach contractions or low blood sugar that control eating, and they seem to eat more because of external cues like the lunch whistle or the attractiveness of food.

And we have hardly begun to describe the complexity of the system for hunger. It is complex because the health maintenance program of the brain controls weight very precisely. Although we may not like it, centers of the brain have pretty much decided for us what our weight will be, and there is less we can do about it consciously than we might wish. We all know people who seem to be able to eat three steaks, fried potatoes, and cheesecake for lunch and have their large meal at dinnertime, all the while having sleek physiques. Others nibble raw carrots once or at most twice during the day and sit down to a nice slice of plain white poached tofu with no sauce in the evening, obscured by a swelling belly. Is it fair? We can't say, but it is the brain which is responsible, and on the average, it is working and managing an optimal health program.

Losing and gaining weight is *not* simply a matter of decreasing calorie intake, because the stabilizing mechanisms of the brain regulate body weight around a set point. There are many means at the brain's disposal to control weight. The hypothalamus can control appetite, and it can control absorption of the food into the body, as well as the metabolic level of the body to change caloric expenditure.

There are many sophisticated ways the brain handles the incoming food. It is not a matter, as was thought, of "calories in and calories out." There is a much more sophisticated system for dealing with intake. Not all calories are equally fattening. Fat in the food leads to more fat deposit in the body since it can be deposited directly in the tissue, while an equal amount of calories of carbohydrates has to be metabolized first and does not contribute as much to deposited fat.

Calories are handled with great precision: Some people get hot, not after seeing another person, but after eating too large a meal. This is because the brain has simply decided that the gorging it has just observed is too much, and it then lights an internal fire, using what is called brown adipose tissue, brown fat to the rest of us. People with a lot of brown fat often sweat it out overnight and return to a good weight in the morning.

It is the brain set point, not conscious decisions, that keeps weight around a predetermined level. We eat about two tons per year, yet our weight usually alters by only a few pounds at most. While a few pounds may seem like a lot to us, consider the remarkable job the brain is doing. Who is counting the calories? It is just about impossible, even for a nutritionist, to consciously regulate food intake to within a few hundred calories a day in order to maintain weight in such a narrow range. The set point (which may be different from the body weight we want) makes it more difficult both to gain and lose weight than we would predict by counting calories.

Some people *are* born to be fat, as their set point is higher. This makes losing weight difficult if not impossible. Fatness is related to the number and size of the adipocites. Obese people have three times the numbers of these fat cells as do people of normal weight. Fat cells are established in the first two years of life. Overfeeding in those years results in an increased number of fat cells. No amount of weight loss after that age lessens the number of fat cells; they remain inside lurking around and waiting patiently to be bloated.

People with excess fat cells have a high set point for food consumption and will continue to be hungry even when their weight is at the supposed "norm." The problem for the "constitutionally heavies" is that their own set point is higher than the cultural norm. They then face two bleak alternatives: constant hunger or being thought of as overweight. They lose and gain weight constantly; their diets do not work. They are fighting a powerful internal biological foe.

The stabilizing mechanisms of the body also serve to discourage weight loss: At the beginning, when one may be high above the real set point, weight loss is easier; as one approaches the set point, however, weight loss is more difficult. This causes many people to go off their diet and return to the original weight. Also, people try to establish a new, lower set point; when this cannot be reached, they abandon all discipline. According to Janet Polivy and Peter Herman, this reaction is known in technical terms as the "what the hell" effect.

The body has a built-in protection against famine that lowers the "set point" drastically when the food supply is low. Then weight loss may be extremely difficult. The limits to which the body can conserve were determined in secret by Jewish doctors in World War II, during the Nazi occupation of Poland. The caloric intake of the residents of the Warsaw Ghetto was decreased by the Nazis from about twenty-four hundred per day to about three hundred; protein intake was cut to about 10 percent of normal.

The record these doctors made of the human body was of an organism struggling heroically to adapt. Body temperature dropped, blood pressure decreased, blood circulated at a slower rate, and the body burned fuel in the most efficient way possible. Only as a last resort was the stored protein in muscles, including the heart, burned. The changes in metabolism to conserve resources undoubtedly saved many lives in the concentration camps, as they probably did when our ancestors were confronted with famine.

In less extreme circumstances deliberately eating less is one means of adjusting weight, but to maintain weight loss, food intake must be continually decreased as the diet goes along, since our caloric needs decrease at lower weight. A diet low enough in calories to decrease weight early in dieting may cause no weight loss or even a weight gain later on. The brain makes a new stabilizing point.

An alternative is to increase exercise, which reduces appetite.

Exercise increases the caloric consumption (heat production) during the exercise. It also increases heat production *after* a meal, and the increase in calories burned during exercise continues during the day. The set point regulation mechanism evolved in a setting in which our ancestors habitually engaged in a moderate amount of physical activity in the course of the day.

The most recent evidence, given wide publicity in the spring of 1986, announced that there are substantial weight benefits for those who walk about twenty-five to thirty miles per week. Exercise seems to reset the set point, something not surprising from our perspective, since this is about the workload that our ancestors adapted to, and is probably the average stabilizing point of the system.

There is a consolation for those never fated to match the ideal of the jeans ads. Remember that the average weight gain is a little below a pound a year for people of average height. This means a man who weighed 165 at thirty will usually weigh 185 or so at sixty. Millions of people gain weight this way; it is the bane of the middle-aged, it is the boon for fitness centers, fad diets, and diet aids. But from the point of view of the brain (and this book) why should this weight gain with age occur? It is for health. It is usually assumed that thin people are healthier—and actuarial tables have been built around this for years. But new research, especially by Reuben Andres, shows that people who are of average weight for their ages (that is, those people who develop the common and typical yearly weight gain) are the healthiest.

Most of the social advice we are given in terms of weight is more likely advice about appearance (look thin = look young) than useful information based on health data. Our brain processes, having evolved over millions of years to adjust weight for health, may well be wiser than our current cultural ideal; so being "overweight" for those people not grossly obese may not be such a losing battle after all.

There are numerous other bodyguards. Some, like the ones we have so far discussed, are reflexive, unconscious, controlled by lower brain structures. Others are more under cortical control and more influenced by social and psychological changes. Later in the book we will explore additional brain mechanisms for minding the body—such as the role of emotions, how beliefs and expectations can promote healing, how the brain talks to the heart and to the immune system, and how pain is regulated through an intrinsic control system.

We need to recognize that the brain is not primarily for educating, speaking, or thinking, but spends the great bulk of its time maintaining the stability of the body, not in preparing for rational discussions or big ideas or for writing music.

The technical term for this maintenance of internal stability is *homeostasis*, meaning a return to *stasis* or a static state. But this term can be misleading. Things are never static within ourselves, or in the outside world; a person's needs change, society changes, growth occurs.

What the brain tries to do is keep the body continuously adapting, and somehow stable, but not static, in a changing world. What is strong enough in youth is not so in maturity; blood supply that is adequate for resting does not suffice for running; metabolic processes which keep the energy supply adequate in winter do not do so in spring. So there are countless systems within the brain orchestrating this rough and always moving stability, as the world changes, as the organism changes, as needs change. We don't yet know how our brain does all of it—we should note that it has taken a long time to perfect these health-maintaining routines—and modern science might still have a bit to learn from them.

We are at the beginning of a new era, one in which the brain's central contribution to resistance to disease is being discovered and enhanced. It has not been done before because medical scientists, like most other human beings, want to tackle problems that are amenable to solutions within a short time. So they typically try to study the simplest systems available.

Bacteria are quite simple. As Salvador Luria once said to one of the authors, "We know everything about them. They move." And understanding these simple structures has paid off enormously.

But the price for such progress has too often been a severe limit on what is acceptable inquiry. Since a small group of researchers sets priorities for funding, it wants to support what is currently understandable. This leads to the conservatisms of science: a set of beliefs that, somehow, the current set of problems is the correct set, even though it might have been selected on the basis of immediate payoff.

It is easy to see why most scientists, brain and medical ones certainly included, have had to limit their inquiry: The understanding of large and complex systems is extremely difficult, given the methods of nineteenth- and early twentieth-century science.

Billions of people make up the earth's population, and their interaction is extremely difficult to measure; this has made hard "scientific" researchers much more comfortable with analysis of simple and small systems.

Just as complex and just as difficult to fathom is the understanding of how the billions of cells in the brain operate, how the brain itself developed, and what it responds to.

In the late 1980s the different research streams about the brain, health, and psychology are beginning to merge. It has taken years of the research work of thousands of scientists to be able to determine the nature of the brain circuitry and communication which enables it to begin to connect such events as the sudden loss of a spouse to the ability of the body to survive infection.

And there is more: Raising hope may increase health, and the attention of friends is an essential part of the brain's "nutrition." Recent discoveries in the endorphin, immune, and cardiovascular systems, combined with new studies of brain physiology, human evolution, and cognitive psychology point to a new understanding of this most mysterious organ.

The brain is the central connection between the different worlds and the different systems that the person lives in.

It connects the output of nerve, muscle, and gland cells together in the body, it generally monitors the operation of all other organ systems, and orchestrates and selects the way information from the outside environment gets inside.

It maintains stability in countless ways. It ultimately controls heartbeat, blood pressure, blood composition and volume, breathing, the entrance of oxygen into the bloodstream, the production, combination, and distribution of thousands of chemicals of the internal pharmacy, the integrity of the internal organs, the safety of the organism, the avoidance of danger, the attachments to family, to friends, and to society, and the creation of mental processes, mental routines, and structures which guide the person safely through immediate and long-term crises.

It is, first and foremost, a healing brain.

CHAPTER THREE

THE SELF-ISH BRAIN:
Feeling Our Way through an Unstable
World

W e don't have a single united brain, but many small brains with their own "small minds." Each piece of the structure evolved and changed to respond to different circumstances. These small minds express different talents and abilities, the capabilities for receiving, processing, constructing, interpreting, and acting upon information from the external and internal worlds. Each small mind is a different mental system, with its own set of rules and priorities. One small system deals with smelling, another with calculating, and still other neural networks with feeling.

This is one reason we have such mixed feelings, mixed motives, and mixed messages, why we do things we don't wish to do, why we act sometimes almost out of our own control, why we are so susceptible to new and exciting events. The new information or the new circumstances shifts the particular small system then operating in the brain, almost like the shift in a multiple personality, and we change much more and are much less consistent than we might have once believed.

That the world is chaotic is fairly easy to credit. That we are so is more difficult, but our mixed nature is the key to understanding why we are at one reckoning so well adapted to the world we live in, and also why changes in one area of information such as beliefs can affect other realms of experience such as internal health. While one could write hundreds of books detailing the brain structures involved in its management of the person and the implications for psychology, we concentrate here on the dominant tendencies of the system: sensing information about changes in the world and judging our situation by feeling.

In the normal course of events, an average human being doesn't need to notice that he or she is ignorant of much of outside reality, that we see only a trillionth of what is out there, that we feel even less, just as we are by design ignorant of the blind spot of our eyes. The brain system is designed to respond to the important events in the outside world, to enable us to survive. It is not designed so that we can have a complete understanding of the world in all its complexity, let alone understand ourselves.

Each organism's sensory system simplifies the world, allowing in those stimuli to which it needs to attend. The cat is a nocturnal animal and so needs its reflective eye, which doubles the incoming light. Insects see infrared radiation, which human beings only feel as warmth, while a frog sees only things that move. Human beings see colors. But there is none of this in truth in the outside world, no infrared "heat," no reflections, no yellow sunsets. Color, heat, and sounds are internal brain processes, not external reality. The brain just gets on with its job in most cases without complex calculation or trouble. Color is given, sound is given, taste is given, pain is given. We have no alternative.

The nerve circuitry feeding into the brain transmits information concerning changes in the external environment; what is important to us are new events: the sun coming up, a sudden loud noise, a change in weather. The sensory systems respond maximally to beginnings and endings of events; they cease responding in between. When an air conditioner is turned on in a room, you notice the hum. Soon you become habituated to the noise. When the machine is turned off, you again take note, this time because of the absence of the noise. The senses are interested in when something new happens.

It is a complicated mess in there, but one which underlies our ability to respond to a few important dimensions of the outside world. Instead of a complete view of the external world which is somehow mirrored within the mind, we strongly select a small part of it and go overboard about it. We possess physical blind spots in the retina, the place where the ganglia feed the nerve circuits to the brain, and we have blind spots at all levels of the nervous system. We have these because of the different kinds of brains within, some of which are specific to different situations, like avoiding certain kinds of food. Some are separate biological centers of specific kinds of ability, like smelling or the recognition of faces. Some of these reflect the general organization of the brain and some are general tendencies of the mind: the need to respond to new events, to search out changes, to compare information and to boil things down to a small point.

Obviously, we don't believe that there are specific detectors which specifically sense social cohesion or the pain of immediate separation or too much stimulation. There *are* hundreds of millions of neural detectors within, which we know about, some specialized for seeing red, for hearing pure tones, for sensing pressure, sugar, salt, and gravity. However, the more complex social events do not have a specific receptor. Instead most immediate impacts are first calculated and their meaning then appraised.

The center point of the internal "commanding self" part of the brain is another primitive action system, one which other forces cannot usually override—emotion. Our view is that the dominant system, the self-ish brain, lies in frontal lobe limbic system linkages. These serve to appraise threats in the environment and organize quick actions. This is not to say that human beings do not have many other "selves" that *can* override the commanding one; actions can be reconsidered, we can learn and grow from experiences, and conscious control can modify ineffective tendencies. But we are saying that most often and most reliably, especially in eras long gone, feeling our way through worked best.

Within the cortex lie separated and large lobes, but each of these lobes, the temporal, parietal, frontal, and occipital, are more important anatomically than functionally. To understand the brain's operations, we have to look at smaller segments of the brain, centers which contain specialized neural systems—talents.

The brain is divided into very many independent and well-defined areas, each of which possesses a rich concentration of certain abilities. In this view, which is becoming more and more established, the brain is seen not as a single organ, but as a collage of different and independent systems, each of which contains component abilities. It has taken the evidence of the past few decades to discern the separate structures which lie almost hidden deep within the brain and which underlie different minds and the different processes within.

In essence, we never operate with a "full deck," but rather with only a small portion of the system live and on the spot at any one time. Different components of the mind are activated and deactivated according to the specific needs of the organism. Consciousness, then, is the complex control system which shifts components in and out, cutting through the enormous amount of information, so that the organism is aware of and responds to essential information.

The "talents" have a wide range, because any organism, especially human beings, have to do many different things at once. Some talents are quite standard abilities, such as the memory for smells; some are high-level, like calculating the trajectory of a comet. The most basic of the talents concern short term survival, the more elaborate concern adapting to the world as it changes, and those still more elaborate concern the thinking abilities and sense of self. There are independent centers of memory, of movement, of mathematical ability, of decoding and producing speech, of sensory analysis, and much more.

We might hope that a rational and judicious component of the human brain controls and orchestrates this parade of talents. Unfortunately for those who hold such a view, but fortunately for the biological survival of the organism, the commanding, controlling mental operating system (which might be called "the self") is much more closely linked with emotions and the system of automatic bodyguards than with conscious thought and reason. The primary job of the brain is to insure survival, not by calculating, plotting, planning, and carefully weighing the alternatives, but by mobilizing the organism to respond quickly to changes, discontinuities, and upsets in the environment, events which might represent threats.

The central readout within ourselves is, therefore, usually an emotional appraisal of a change in the outside environment: Is it harmful? should I move toward it or not? Should I stop or change what I am doing? Is it surprising? Should I attack? To insure a rapid response to these appraisals, the self is linked with certain automatic response patterns, emotions, which prepare us for action. While there is much more to emotions than a simple positive negative, stop/start, approach/avoid program, more of our lives is determined by these primitive appraisals than we, the conscious thinkers, might believe. It is because the system worked well before human beings appeared and survived the move of Ghana far away from Georgia. It has been around a long time, and we have to work through it in almost all normal activities.

Information about the inside and outside world and plans and controls are all assembled by a most uniquely human talent—a system concerned with the maintenance of the individual self. While we do not believe that one should try to locate the locus in the brain of the self, many of the functions of this system are probably dependent upon the decisions carried out within the frontal lobes of both of the cerebral hemispheres.

The frontal lobes are a crossroads: They lie at the intersection of the neural pathways that convey information from the parietal areas of the brain about other people and events in the world and information from the limbic system about one's own state, and they also contribute to the control of basic systems like heart rate. They are so richly connected to the limbic system that many neuroanatomists classify the frontal lobes as a part of them. Certainly there are different forms of emotions represented within each of the lobes, as well as some control of the expression of emotions. In tragic cases, damage to the frontal areas results in the inability to carry out plans, to know on a long-term basis who one is.

The first recorded, and still the most famous, case of such damage was that of a railroad worker named Phineas Gage, who in 1868 had a piece of the rail line permanently embedded in his skull, but survived. He lived, but his personality and sense of self disappeared.

> His physical health is good, and I am inclined to say that he has recovered. . . . The equilibrium or balance, so to speak, between his intellectual faculty and animal propensities, seems to have been destroyed. He is fitful, irreverent, indulging at times in the grossest profanity (which was not previously his custom), manifesting but little deference for his fellows, impatient of restraint or advice when it conflicts with his desires, at times pertinaciously obstinate, yet capricious and vacillating, devising many plans of future operation, which are no sooner arranged than they are abandoned in turn for others appearing more feasible. A child in his intellectual capacity and manifestations, he has the animal passions of a strong man. Previous to his injury, though untrained in the schools, he possessed

a well-balanced mind, and was looked upon by those who knew him as a shrewd, smart business man, very energetic and persistent in executing all his plans of operation. In this regard, his mind was radically changed, so decidedly that his friends and acquaintances said he was "no longer Gage."

The cortex of human beings is divided into two separate hemispheres, each of which is specialized for different functions, different abilities, and styles of thought: verbal and spatial thinking. Analyzing information sequentially and simultaneously seem to be the special functions of the left and right sides of the brain, respectively. But evidence is also accumulating that different emotions seem to involve the frontal lobes of the two different hemispheres.

When one of us, Robert Ornstein, was beginning his studies of the functions of the two hemispheres, one of the consistent puzzles came from some Italian studies in which the hemispheres were disabled. These studies were typically done upon depressed patients who were given electric shock to one hemisphere or another.

With the left hemisphere knocked out, the patients had what the Italian neurologists called a "catastrophic" reaction; they wailed and acted as if they had lost their spouses and cried out until the effect wore off. With the right hemisphere out, it was almost opposite; they seemed happy. Many, if not most, of the researchers found the evidence easy to ignore, and so work went on studying the effects of different kinds of thinking.

In 1970 Robert Ornstein and his colleague David Galin developed a method in which the electrical potentials from the brain could be compared between the two hemispheres. These voltages, about twenty to thirty millionths of a volt, appear on the scalp and can be picked up by an electroencephalograph (EEG). With this method, different kinds of thinking could be compared with different brain activity. When a person was writing a letter the left hemisphere was active, the right more idling. This pattern reversed with spatial and intuitive thoughts.

Richard Davidson, then of the State University of New York at Purchase, extended this method to study the brain representation of emotions. He recorded from the two frontal areas of the brain while stimulating and encouraging different kinds of feelings. He asked his subjects to relive the angriest episode of their lives or the happiest. He also showed different kinds of emotional information to the two hemispheres, using a tachistoscope, which can flash slides to one half of the visual field.

The nerves from the right half of each eye go to the right side of the brain (and receive information from the left half of space) and vice versa. In one experiment with Reuter-Lorenz, Davidson asked people to indicate which of two faces showed the strongest feeling. Two faces, one neutral and one either happy or sad, were presented, one in each visual field. When one of the two faces was happy, subjects were faster at recognizing it when it appeared in the right visual field. Conversely, when one of the faces was sad, response times were faster when the sad face was in the left visual field.

The right hemisphere recognizes sadness faster, the left happiness. The results are consistent and quite important: On EEG and recognition measures, emotions like anger and sadness involve the right hemisphere more than the left, while emotions like happiness involve the left hemisphere. Davidson has even found that very young babies already respond to different emotions differently within their two frontal lobes.

Why do we have such separated emotions; why are they divided in the brain? Of course no one knows, but many investigators believe that it has to do with the way different emotions mobilize the body. The two hemispheres are thought by many neuropsychologists to possess different forms of muscle control. The right seems to have more control of the large motor programs, which move the great muscles of the limbs, and the left seems to be involved in the smaller muscle movements, which control, for instance, finger dexterity. So if running were controlled by one specific neural system, it would make more sense to put the emotions that are associated with running and moving the arms, fighting or fleeing in the same area of the brain.

The current general understanding is that the right hemisphere's control over the large muscle systems allows us to move quickly and to avoid trouble, while the left hemisphere's control over the small muscle system allows us to approach things we are happy about. Think about how your muscles would respond (on the one hand) to a threat or (on the other hand) to the sight of a loved one. The feelings and the motor control are perhaps lined up in the brain. We may have different positive and negative self-emotion systems, which divide control of many behaviors.

Consider the happiness we derive from sweets. The pleasure derived from sweet-tasting foods encourages us to search for more sweet things to eat using fine motor movements activated by the left hemisphere—more involved, it seems, in happy feelings than the right. Our sweet tooth had adaptive value in our evolutionary history because sweet fruits were more nutritious and unlikely to be poisonous. In a colorful passage, the psychologist Silvan Tomkins wrote, "If, instead of pain, we had an orgasm to injury, we would be destined to bleed to death."

But negative emotions have a different information value: They are probably intermediate between the registration of a change in the outside world and the activation message to "do something" within. In this view, positive feelings are read internally as an automatic signal to continue to do what we are doing, while negative feelings are more urgent and signal that something should be taken care of. But of course this is not all there is to emotions—they are not merely "good," "bad," "stop," or "go" systems.

Like the weight regulation program, conscious decisions about what to do in many different circumstances have probably not been sufficient. Emotions signal that something important is happening. An animal that becomes fearful and excited about an approaching attacker is readier to respond and to defend itself. A human who experiences sexual love is more likely to reproduce than one who does not. An enraged organism is prepared to attack; a fearful one is prepared to flee; a joyous one is willing and eager.

Emotions not only initiate and direct action but *sustain* and engage action; when you are afraid, you will probably run longer and faster than if you are bored. This is a reaction that is certainly useful in avoiding danger. Coaches recognize this by giving pre-game pep talks, making the team "emotionally involved." The description athletes use is "pumped up," one case in which slang is quite accurate.

Feelings are automatic and involuntary: When frightened we are almost automatically "primed" to run or to defend ourselves. You may decide to be expressionless when someone embarrasses you, but your blush may give you away. To borrow from e. e. cummings: "Feeling is first." We get angry and embarrassed often when we do not want to or fall in love almost by accident. Emotions are similar among all peoples of the world, and even between humans and other animals; they comprise relatively automatic patterns of responding to different situations.

They simplify experience by preparing us for action. We are not sure that "something has to tell us what is important" is the right way to describe it, but some system, within the warring separate ones of the brain, has to seize priority when there is trouble, when there is a storm, a fistfight, or difficulties in work. We have to remember important moments. We have to act and move our large muscles fast when there is a threat. We may also move slowly toward something, using our fine motor movements when there is something in our field which is pleasing. We don't caress by jerking our shoulders.

Emotions are a pretty standard part of the human nervous system's program. Charles Darwin observed that all peoples of the world, from an Oxford don to an aborigine, express grief by contracting their facial muscles in the same way. This is true of the other emotions as well. In rage, the lips are retracted and teeth clenched. There are similarities in the snarl and in disgust. All over the world, flirting is signaled by a lowering of the eyelids or the head, followed by direct eye contact. Embarrassed people all over the world close their eyes, turn their heads away or cover their faces. And anger is recognizable in all cultures.

The German ethologist Eibl-Eibesfeldt filmed children born deaf and blind and found that basic facial expressions—smiling, laughing, pouting, crying, those of surprise and of anger—occurred in appropriate situations. Blind children show the same pattern of development of smiling as sighted children with the difference that social smiling becomes increasingly responsive to the mother's voice and touch instead of to her face. In humans, emotions are primarily expressed in the face.

The facial musculature of most animals below mammals does not permit much more than the opening and closing of the mouth and eyes. Mammals, especially primates and humans, have more complicated patterns of muscles that allow a variety of facial expressions. In addition, because gorillas, chimpanzees, and humans have a more upright posture, their faces are much more conspicuous to others than those of lower animals. There is also increasing frontal orientation of the eyes and, in humans, stereoscopic vision, which leads to sharper focus on other animals' faces. Facial hair is relatively lacking in humans and is further accentuated by the framing of head hair. The face is the primary organ of human social communication, although other body gestures, such as movement of hands and feet, are also important and are currently being investigated.

Although emotions may be judged by facial expressions, many of the emotional reactions themselves involve arousal of the autonomic nervous system. Interestingly, the actual bodily response pattern in emotions matches quite closely the colloquial expressions: "My heart leaped when I saw her"; "I've got butterflies in my stomach." The cardiovascular and gastrointestinal systems are involved in most emotional reactions and embody the emergency arousal in the sympathetic nervous system or its opposite, withdrawal.

Two emergency systems evolved long before humanity. One, which Walter Cannon called "flight or fight," involves mobilization of resources for massive motor activity to deal with threat or danger; the other, "conservation-withdrawal," produces inactivity and conserves energy to reduce threats and to render the organism less conspicuous to its enemies. In some cases an animal will appear dead to the aggressor, who then ceases the attack and moves on. The winter hibernation of the bear is an extreme form of conservation-withdrawal.

Each of these patterns has its own neural organization. The flight-or-fight emergency system prepares for action by increases in skeletal muscle tone and sympathetic nervous system activity. The rate and the strength of the heartbeat increase, allowing oxygen to be pumped more rapidly into the cells of the muscles. The liver releases stored sugar for the use of the muscles. The blood supply shifts from the skin and viscera to irrigate the muscles and brain. Respiration quickens. The blood's ability to seal wounds is increased. We are ready to move in any direction, to hit with maximum strength, or to run as quickly as possible.

Conservation-withdrawal increases the body's isolation—it decreases muscle tone, increases parasympathetic activity, and slows down metabolic processes and oxygenation. In the normal course of events there is a stability: When one of these systems becomes more active the other becomes inhibited, and high levels of activation of one inhibit the other completely. One rarely takes a nap in the middle of a fight, and bears, for instance, do not often strike out at passing animals while deep within their winter hibernation.

The sympathetic system prepares the internal organs for emergencies, when there are extra demands on the body. It operates "in sympathy" with the emotions, like an accelerator pedal on a car, telling the body to go. The signs of sympathetic activation are sweating and other symptoms of arousal. The sympathetic nervous system is usually activated by the unusual: Emergencies, ecstasy, excitement.

The parasympathetic system is more conservative. It acts like a brake on the sympathetic system and returns the body to normal after an emergency. Typically, when an exciting event has passed, heart rate slows and dryness of the mouth begins to abate because the parasympathetic system actively slows heart rate and deactivates certain internal organs.

The two kinds of signals, "go" and "slow down," are carried by different nerve circuits, and the messages are carried by different neurotransmitters. Norepinephrine carries the sympathetic message, acetylcholine the parasympathetic message. The sympathetic neurons are centralized in the brain, acting on their target from a distance. The parasympathetic system is decentralized; each ganglion (collection of nerve cell bodies) is located near the organ it serves.

The major physiological effect of emotion is activation. Emotions turn on (activate) the body's emergency reaction, allowing us to prepare for immediate action. Very many of the reactions involved in emotions involve the activating mechanisms of the sympathetic nervous system. Underlying most strong feelings— anger, fear, joy—are the following: An increase in the secretion of norepinephrine in the bloodstream by the adrenals activates the internal organs; and heart rate, blood pressure, and blood volume increase, allowing more blood to flow to the muscles and the face. We are "flushed with excitement." Skin resistance, salivation, and gastric motility decrease; respiration, sweating, and pupil size increase.

That many emotions are grossly similar in their activating capacity (compare the face of a beauty contest winner upon learning she has won with a similar woman grieving) has caused many scientists to think the go–no go system is the only important aspect of emotions, and that all brain and bodily signs are alike. This is too much of an oversimplification.

Fear and happiness do feel different, and so do anger and joy. It seems only logical that different emotions would cause quite different bodily reactions. In a recent and important series of studies, our colleague Paul Ekman of the University of California at San Francisco has shown that we can call up different emotions within, using only simple poses of the face, somewhat like Method acting. In these studies Ekman asked people to assume different facial expressions, like raising the eyebrows and lowering the lips. When they did, they *felt* different emotions, such as anger and happiness. Ekman was able to record that consistently different patterns of autonomic nervous system activity characterized different emotions, especially anger. Perhaps people can begin to learn to control their emotions using deliberate techniques. This, as one can easily see, could have great effects on health.

Also, different people seem to show *different* characteristic "emotional" responses to situations. One person may become flushed with anger as well as joy, another may sweat, a third may have stomach reactions.

In studies of people who experience the same emotion, the pattern of activation is different. In one study of students' anxiety regarding an examination, some sweated while others' heartbeats increased. However, all other individual differences involve specific components of the emergency reaction of the sympathetic division of the autonomic nervous system (ANS). The only specific body pattern that consistently relates to various people's emotional expressions is facial expression.

There are standard emotions, common to all of those with a human brain. Fear is an immediate and specific emotional reaction to a specific threatening stimulus. Young birds show fear if the shadow of a hawk—even a wooden one—passes over them. However, as we go up the phylogenetic scale, fear may become highly symbolic and/or more future-oriented than immediate— anxiety rather than fear.

Anxiety is a more generalized reaction and develops in response to the anticipation that something harmful *may* occur in the future. This harm may not be just physical but also psychological, as in a threat to a person's self-esteem. The stimulus for fear is usually clear and immediate, but when a situation is ambiguous and the person is not sure what is going to occur, he or she may feel a vague sense of apprehension and become anxious.

These "stress emotions," while unpleasant at the moment, usually alert a person to the fact that something is (potentially) wrong, and that action may be necessary. For example, an executive who is slightly anxious about an upcoming meeting is likely to prepare more than one who does not particularly care about it and is not anxious. Healthy fear may keep someone from walking alone at night in dangerous sections of town. However, when emotional reactions become too great, they disrupt stability. The executive may be too anxious to do a good job, or a person may become too afraid to leave the house even during the daytime.

There are modern difficulties with our prepared emotional selves. A basic emotional reaction such as fear is probably innate, a shortcut to action. In the long course of evolution emotions probably evolved to match well the needs of most organisms. Fear of snakes, for instance, probably saved many lives. However, the situation in human beings is different: The dangers of the modern world are unprecedented in our evolutionary history. The fear of nuclear war, for instance, is not as palpable as fear of snakes: There is no identifiable stimulus, no obvious and immediate course of action. The *meaning* of a situation and its appraisal are major factors in human emotional life.

We appraise along fixed lines of inference: Is it good or bad, benign or threatening? alive/dead, strong/weak, fast/slow, active/ passive? Charles Osgood, who proposed these dimensions of emotions, describes their value:

> What is important to us now, as it was way back in the age of Neanderthal Man, about the sign of a thing is: First, does it refer to something *good* or *bad* for me (is it an antelope or a saber-toothed tiger)? Second, does it refer to something that is *strong* or *weak* with respect to me (saber-toothed tiger, or a mosquito)? And third, for behavioral purposes, does it refer to something which is *active* or *passive* (is it a saber-toothed tiger or merely a pool of quicksand, which I can simply walk around)?

Feelings change as new information comes in. One night, as David Sobel relates, he awakened to the sound of a strange noise upstairs in his house:

> I was aroused, fearful. Eyes wide open. Muscles tense. Heart pounding. What could the sound be? Did I lock the door? A burglar? A squirrel? Was the roof falling? With each thought I was prepared to act differently. Then I remembered that a friend of mine from out of town had asked to stay over. He must have noticed that I was

asleep and then let himself in. Once I realized what had happened, I went back to sleep.

It may be that the question, "Which comes first, emotions or cognitions?" is like asking about the chicken and egg. It is perhaps more profitable to view emotions and thoughts as part of a feedback system in which each influences the other and appraisals are followed by reappraisals. Sometimes emotional evaluation may come first: "I like wine" is an evaluation. But sometimes the evaluation may well come after a long analysis: "I don't like this white wine after all; it's too sweet."

Feelings are perhaps the most central readout in the brain, and the self-system involving decision centers in the frontal lobes probably influence every brain process. They may cause us to seek out different information, remember differently, think and evaluate differently. They also cause health problems, among them cancer and sudden heart attacks, which we will discuss later.

How we express feelings seems to influence health. Lieberman found that the single most successful prediction for long life in aged individuals was how much aggressiveness they expressed and how much anger. Passivity and refusal to express anger may well lead, as many people think, to a biological deterioration or it may heighten the magnitude of the stress that someone experiences. Aggressive behavior in some circumstances seems to enhance survival. The individuals who are most likely to survive are those who are "aggressive, irritating, narcissistic and demanding . . . being a good guy—having qualities associated with passive acceptance—was a trait . . . found in old people not likely to survive the crises of environmental changes."

The aggressive individuals seemed to be more likely to have a realistic appraisal of threats and were less likely to deny their real emotional impact. However, there is not a simple story here: It is not good to be not nice, and it is not always good to be nice. Hostility seems, on the basis of much evidence, to be bad for the heart, and we shall discuss this later.

We have special access to our own choices, so we assume that our own conscious decisions have a superior place in the scheme of things and are fundamentally different from lower-level "automatic processes." But conscious mental processes use the same chemicals, and most of the same neural systems, as other systems which run the body. These lower level systems, concerned primarily with the integrity and maintenance of the self, probably have the commanding role in our makeup.

The emotions are most often the internal readout of what action to take. Sometimes health will suffer from the exercise of short-term emotions like anger; sometimes the organism benefits from a threat defused. The lines between mind, brain, and self and the rest of society are not clear in truth, not as clear as we might like to think. It is not that mind and body are being united, but that we are finally getting away from our oversimplified conceptions of their difference.

We have a brain which operates much more with emotions in mind than reason. This may have served our ancestors well when they were faced with threats like a charging wild animal. The emotions elicit a highly adaptive emergency reaction preparing the organism for flight or fight. Hardly any physiological process is not affected by this massive mobilization.

This primitive flight-or-fight response continues to operate within us, but does so now when we are stuck in traffic jams, facing shocking tax bills, or confronting a contrary boss. Our bodies automatically prepare to flee or fight, but, all too often, neither response is appropriate. Persistent, repeated elicitation of this inappropriate response disrupts nearly every bodily system influencing immune disorders, heart disease, gastrointestinal disease and hypertension. What we need to develop is an understanding of which aspects of brain control are fixed, and which can be changed to suit modern times, so that we can adjust the innate health-maintaining powers of our brain to suit current conditions.

Happily the legacy of our brain's evolution provides us with ample evidence that powerful brain mechanisms can be mobilized to protect and restore health. Since the brain is continually shifting priorities and operating systems, cultivating or suggesting certain beliefs to a receptive brain can cause profound shifts in mental and physiological functioning. When a belief is brought into consciousness it brings up a whole host of associated processes, as when you turn a light on in a corner of a room and illuminate many things which were previously invisible.

Events and ideas, as well as large systems of mind, constantly

wheel in and out of consciousness, shifting from moment to moment almost chaotically from one operating system to another.
We shift from one idea to another since our brain processes are
surprisingly inconsistent and unstable. This is why a belief or an
assumption about reality can have such an effect: It shifts the
piece of mind that is operating at the time.

The potential to manipulate the mind in order to foster healing
has not gone unnoticed. Through the millennia, observant people
have found that certain beliefs, certain casts of mind like expectant faith, elicit healing consequences, even though they may not
make rational sense. We send flowers to the sick at the hospital.
Why?

Beyond Belief

CHAPTER FOUR

THE POWERFUL PLACEBO

*S*ir William Osler was already a famous physician in the early years of the twentieth century. His contributions to medicine were so important that a large section of the *Journal of the American Medical Association* issue of December 22, 1969, was devoted to him. In this issue of *JAMA*, Patrick Mallam, an Oxford physician, recounted the treatment by Osler of his three-year-old brother in 1906. The boy was quite ill, probably dying, from disorders common at the time.

One remembers a young brother with very severe whooping-cough and bronchitis, unable to eat and wholly irresponsive to the blandishments of parents and devoted nurses alike. Clinically it was not an abstruse case, but [medical] weapons were few and recovery seemed unlikely. The Regius [Osler], about to present for degrees and hard pressed for time, arrived already wearing his doctor's robes. To a small child this was the advent of a doctor, if doctor in fact it was, from quite a different planet. It was more probably Father Christmas.

After a very brief examination this unusual visitor sat down, peeled a peach, sugared it and cut it into pieces. He then presented it bit by bit with a fork to the entranced patient, telling him to eat it up, and that he would not be sick but would find it did him good as it was a most special fruit. Such proved to be the case. As he hurried off, Osler, *most uncharacteristically*, patted my father kindly on the back and said with deep concern, "I'm sorry Ernest but I don't think I shall see the boy again, there's very little chance when they're as bad as that." Happily events turned out otherwise, and for the next forty days this constantly busy man came to see the child, and for each of these forty days he put on his doctor's robes in the hall before going into the sick room.

After some two or three days, recovery began to be obvious and the small boy always ate or drank and retained some nourishment which Osler gave him with his own two hands. If the value of personal approach, the quick turning to effect of an accidental psychological advantage (in this case decor) the consideration and extra trouble required to meet the needs of an individual patient, were ever illustrated, here it was in its fullest flower. It would, I submit, be impossible to find a fairer example of healing as an art. This kind of inspired magic, independent of higher degrees and laboratory gimmicks is given only to a doctor with a real vocation, and the will to employ it.

There are many reasons why we chose this incident to begin this section of the book. Dr. William Osler, or "Billy O" in the commemoration volume of the *Journal* just cited, was the most influential and important physician of the nineteenth- and early twentieth-centuries. This story shows well how Osler could use the ritual trappings of the profession, such as his status and his magnificent scarlet robe, as well as the peach, to produce an effect in his young hopeless patient. We also have Dr. Patrick Mallam's thoughtful description, from the viewpoint of both a physician and an older brother. And the last reason is that the boy, Jack Mallam, lived and continues to live a long and happy life, and also went on to father the wife of one of the authors of this book, Robert Ornstein.

But Oxford is not unusual, as nearly every society has its sacred shrine, a place to which sick people flock with the expectation of healing and improved health. The central features of religious shrines which mobilize the expectant faith of the pilgrims can be easily identified. The shrine is typically an impressive structure presided over by a hierarchical priesthood. The priests undergo arduous training and perform arcane rituals to invoke the healing deities to come to the aid of the ailing pilgrim. The community is mobilized in support of a sick person, who is encouraged to feel cared for and hopeful about the future.

Consider Lourdes, the most famous of Western religious healing shrines. Each year more than 2 million pilgrims are drawn to the healing spring where in 1858 Marie-Bernarde Soubirous (Saint Bernadette) had her vision. Thousands of the pilgrims are chronically ill, and, having failed to find effective medical treatment, turn to the shrine as a last resort.

Even before arriving at the shrine, the ailing pilgrim's hopes are mobilized by the elaborate preparation: the collection of funds for the journey, the medical examinations, the making of travel plans for the pilgrim and the patient's family.

Our own healing shrines celebrate the religion of *Our Lady of the Single Germ and High-Tech Medical Science.* All the technology which dominates the modern hospital carries a symbolic meaning in addition to its technical function. Psychiatrist Jerome Frank of Johns Hopkins School of Medicine describes the modern hospital as a healing shrine in this way:

> Let us imagine, if you will, how a great teaching hospital might look to an anthropologist from Mars who is studying healing shrines in America. He would learn that the hospital has a reputation as a site of amazing cures, and eventually would ferret out the chaplain's office and the chapel, tangible vestiges of a belief system still widely held but clearly secondary to the faith in Science.
>
> He would learn that the shrine's servants are organized into many echelons, each having its own insignia of rank and function. The priesthood and priests in training communicate in a special language, unintelligible to the layman, and prominently display on their person healing amulets and charms, such as reflex hammers, stethoscopes and ophthalmoscopes. At the lowest level are the postulants in their short white jackets; above them the acolytes, who wear white suits; and above them the high priests, especially impressive in their long, white, starched coats. All are expected to dedicate themselves to the service of the shrine, regardless of personal hardships or interference with connubial felicity and other satisfactions of life.
>
> Turning to the architectural structure, he would probably be impressed with the massive labyrinthine buildings, through whose many orifices pilgrims seeking health are continually streaming. Inside he would find a complex series of chambers, certain of which are open to the uninitiated, such as the wards, while members of the staff alone have access to others where they perform arcane healing rituals, such as laboratories, operating rooms, radiotherapy rooms and intensive care units. These rooms contain spectacular machines that beep and gurgle and flash lights or emit immensely powerful but invisible rays, thereby impressively invoking the healing powers

of Science. The operating rooms are the holy of holies where the most dramatic and difficult healing rituals are conducted and which even the priests can enter only after donning special costumes and undergoing purification rites known as "scrubbing." So jealously guarded are the mysteries of the operating rooms that patients are rendered unconscious before entering them.

In short, all medical and surgical procedures conducted within the walls of a hospital, although viewed as purely scientific by the staff, may in addition mobilize something else, sometimes called "the faith that heals." Despite their emphasis on the technology of healing, hospitals still carry the aura of healing shrines in the eyes of many, if not most, of their patients.

Perhaps one of the most tangible symbols of the healing power of the doctor is the pill. In addition to whatever specific pharmacological activity the medication might have, the giving and taking of medication is a cue which often triggers a positive response. The belief of the patient and doctor in the power of the medication or treatment has historically been one of the most potent therapeutic agents, often derided as "just a placebo." But let us consider placebos for a moment.

Purging, puking.

Cupping, cutting.

Blistering and bleeding.

Sweating and shocking.

Freezing and frying.

Throughout medical history the real heroes have been those patients who have submitted to and endured the bizarre and untested treatments offered in the name of medical science. Potions of powdered mummies, frog sperm, lizard tongues, unicorn horns, and animal dung have been offered to people under the name of "medicine." It is obvious why frogs would be quite interested in their sperm, less so why you and we might.

At the turn of the century the prominent physician Oliver Wendell Holmes said that if all the drugs available were tossed into the ocean, it would be all the better for mankind and all the worse for the fishes. Yet in spite of the patently useless and quite often dangerous treatments offered throughout medical history, people seemed to get better.

If they had not done so, the institution of medicine would not have survived. That it did survive for thousands of years with so few viable treatments suggests that the most important component of the healing process is, and has always been, something resident within the patient himself. Our heroic patient did not believe that he was being healed by the abilities within and was encouraged to attribute the "cures" to the authority figure in charge, so despite the toxic and worse effects of such treatments, fraudulent healers and ineffective physicians were revered for centuries.

Now, there are many reasons why those who are stricken ill become well. The first is that most ailments are "self-limited." If a doctor does nothing or merely tells the patient to take two aspirin or two frog-sperm pellets, the chances are fair that the patient will feel better in the morning, or at some time later, during the course of most illnesses.

Many illnesses follow their own specific "natural history," and people are most likely to seek help at the worst point—if graphed, this would be the low point on the curve. Then, when they improve, they naturally attribute their improvement to the treatment they have received.

The second reason is that the unlikely remedies did contain some physiologically active ingredients. Leeches used in the medieval practices of bloodletting contain, by modern chemical analysis, at least four specifically active biochemical substances that counter different diseases. However, most of the remedies in the long history of medicine were probably much less effective than leeches.

Medicine has not actually had such a great run: Most discoveries throughout medical history have actually been unexplained by the usual canons of medicine. It was not in most cases the specific medical remedy that usually cured the patient. It was the *belief* in the remedy and in the healer (or in something else) that seems to have mobilized powerful innate self-healing mechanisms within the brain.

The long history of medical treatment is, for the overwhelming part, a history of how strong belief heals.

But how can positive emotions, positive feelings, states of expectancy, hope, and wishful thinking in themselves promote healing or staying healthy in the face of disease?

There is promising evidence in what has been usually termed the "placebo effect," which refers to sugar pills, pills that are or are apparently chemically inert, or to any procedure or any therapy for which there is no specific physiological activity relevant to the condition being treated.

The word *placebo* itself comes from the Latin, meaning "I shall please," and the implications are intriguing. Does this refer to the doctor or healer giving something to please or to placate the patient even though the medicine has no specific pharmacological activity for the ailment? Does it refer to the patient's own decision to get better, possibly in order to please the doctor, so that the healer will not feel his or her efforts have gone for naught?

In either case, the placebo has been viewed within the medical research community largely as a nuisance, as something to be shunted aside and ignored, "controlled *for*" rather than thought of as something to be understood in its own right. It is common for authors in a report on a new drug to take pains to show that its effect cannot be accounted for by the placebo effect alone.

But these methodological refinements, useful as they are, allow us to continue to ignore the importance of the "placebo" itself. For example, in the evaluation of a medication for treatment of peptic ulcer disease, the experimental drug may be found to be 20 percent more effective than the placebo, curing, say 50 to 60 percent. However, the fact that the placebo relieved symptoms in 30 to 40 percent of patients may pass without comment. A parallel may make this clear. Our current attitude to the placebo is like our previous attitude toward penicillin. The mold from which penicillin is derived was considered a "contaminant" that interfered with the results of many important biological and medical experiments.

Penicillin was treated as a contaminant until it was noted that the mold had some special properties *itself*; it inhibited the growth of bacteria. Only then was the mold which led to the modern wonder drugs investigated and its power for healing put to use. Similarly, the placebo deserves to be regarded as a potent therapeutic intervention in its own right. Understanding how the placebo effect works may well reveal the means to strengthen the innate healing systems of the body.

Placebos have a profound effect on a very wide range of disorders. In 1955 Henry Beecher of the Harvard Medical School reviewed a large number of studies and found that, on average, a third of the people who were given placebos reported satisfactory relief of their symptoms. To give you an idea of the range of effects, the symptoms included: postoperative wound pain; seasickness; headaches; coughs; anxiety and other disorders of nervousness.

Subsequent studies have only added to the picture: improvements in high blood pressure; angina; depression; acne; asthma; hay fever; colds; insomnia; arthritis; ulcers; gastric acidity; migraine; constipation; obesity; blood counts; lipoprotein levels; and more. If such a treatment suddenly became available, we would believe that we have discovered a new wonder drug comparable to penicillin. Moreover, no system of the body appears immune to the effect.

The effect of placebos can be more potent than expected drug effects. In one case, it produced a result directly opposite to that of the drug which was being used. Consider a series of experiments with a woman suffering from severe nausea and vomiting. Nothing her doctors gave her seemed to help. Objective measurement of her gastric contractions showed a disrupted pattern consistent with the severe nausea she reported. The doctors then offered her a "new and extremely powerful wonder drug" which would, they said, unquestionably cure her nausea. Within twenty minutes of taking this new drug her nausea disappeared, and the same objective gastric tests now read normal.

The drug she was given was not, of course, a new drug designed to relieve nausea. It was syrup of ipecac, which is generally used to *induce* vomiting. In this case the placebo effect associated with the suggestion that the drug would relieve vomiting was powerful enough to counteract the direct and opposite pharmacological action of the drug itself. The syrup of ipecac when presented with the strong suggestion of relief of nausea acted as a cue to the brain which triggered a series of self-regulatory responses.

Not all the results of placebos are positive and therapeutic. An entire range of symptoms including palpitations, drowsiness, and headaches as well as diarrhea and nausea can be produced by placebos.

One classic experiment was performed on medical students in a pharmacology class. The professor lectured about stimulant and sedative medication, describing in detail the effects each has on the body and the side effects which might be anticipated with each. The students took either a pink pill, "the stimulant," or a blue pill, "the depressant," and recorded each other's symptoms, blood pressure, and heart rate.

About half the students experienced specific and measurable physiological reactions such as decreased blood pressure and heart rate as well as dizziness, watery eyes, abdominal pain, and the like. All the symptoms were consistent with the drug taken, either the stimulant or the depressant. But of course the students were given inert pills, whose color, coupled with the students' expectations, produced the effects.

This is the standard kind of placebo study and is widely reported. But the placebo effect is an important part of *every* therapeutic procedure. Surgery provides an especially impressive example. In the mid-1950s a new surgical procedure was introduced to provide relief from the symptoms of chest pain due to coronary heart disease. The procedure was called "internal mammary ligation" and involved tying off an artery in the chest.

In the early evaluations performed by the understandably enthusiastic surgeons, about 40 percent of the patients reported improvement in chest pain while 65 to 75 percent reported considerable improvement. There were also hopeful reports of increased exercise tolerance and improvements on the electrocardiogram. A rush of operations followed.

But despite all the enthusiasm many surgeons doubted the physiological basis of the treatment. Two groups of skeptics decided to carry out an important test of the surgery. You will see why we highlight this study, for it would be impossible to do today, and it reveals much about the powerful placebo component, probably present in all surgery.

Patients who were candidates for the artery-tying operation were randomly assigned to receive either that operation or a sham operation. In both cases an incision was made in the chest. But one group had their arteries tied, and the other was simply closed up with no therapeutic procedure—a complete placebo operation.

So here is quite a good test. Imagine it: You are wheeled into the operating room, given a general anesthetic, your chest is cut and then closed up, you go through the postoperative pain, drugs, and any complications. But you have not been given any specific treatment!

The benefits from this placebo surgery were as great as the artery-tying operation.

The operation was finally abandoned but not until more than 10,000 operations had been performed.

We can't do this kind of research deliberately any more due to the restrictions placed on what we can do to human subjects. But the effects of positive expectancy in surgery are still apparent in a newer surgical procedure, called coronary artery bypass grafting. In this operation, diseased sections of the arteries which feed the heart are bypassed with a new vein created from grafts taken from veins in the patient's legs. Initially, this surgical procedure was highly successful, with over 90 percent of patients reporting improvement in symptoms, and 75 percent of patients doing better on exercise stress tests.

But a cold look at the evidence is different: Of those who claimed they felt better only about 20 percent showed actual improvement of heart function when tested, 60 percent showed no improvement, and 20 percent were even worse following the operation.

How do we account for the improvement in symptoms in the absence of corresponding improvement in the function of the heart? Consider the tremendous forces at work to engender a state of positive expectancy in the patient. The patient arrives on the surgeon's doorstep suffering from terrifying, if not life-threatening, symptoms.

An operation is offered as the last hope. The surgeon explains to the patient the rationale for the procedure and reinforces their shared belief system on how the operation will improve blood flow to the oxygen-deprived heart muscle. The patient undergoes a series of preparatory tests to determine whether he is a "candidate" for the surgery.

The inner workings of the heart are thence revealed to the patient through an impressive array of technological gadgetry. The whole procedure builds to a climax, an impressive and expensive display of the miracle of modern medicine. The patient is cut open, his heart stopped, repaired, and then started again. Few faith healers or shamans can mount such a dramatic performance of healing power. How could the patient fail to improve after all that?

Means by which the placebo effect can take place range from leeches to heart surgery, from potions to pills. But what governs whether a placebo will work and who will respond? The final common pathway for the placebo is the belief in the remedy and expectation of improvement. A German physician named Rheder attempted a form of clinical trial on three patients in the hospital: One had chronic gall bladder disease; one had severe pancreatitis, with accompanying weight loss, constipation, and depression; and the third had inoperable cancer of the uterus, with a massive collection of fluid in her abdomen, anemia, and profound weakness.

Rheder visited a faith healer in the neighborhood who practiced absent healing and asked him to attempt to treat his three patients. He supplied the necessary information about them, and the healer tried during twelve sessions in the following few weeks to project a healing force to the patients. Rheder did not tell the patients what was happening, but he and his associates monitored them carefully for any significant change in their clinical condition over the next few weeks. There was none.

When the healer was no longer working on the cases, Rheder then told the patients he had located a very powerful healer who was prepared to project his healing energy for them at such and such a time on such and such days. He made it clear that the healer had the reputation of successfully healing many like themselves, and by the appointed time of the healing each patient "most longingly" expected to be cured.

Within a few days of the appointed "healing" time the patient with chronic gall bladder disease became free of pain and remained symptom-free for a year. The patient with pancreatitis had restoration of normal bowel function, was able to leave her bed, and gained thirty pounds. The patient with inoperable cancer of the uterus experienced a decrease in swelling and fluid in her abdomen, an increase in appetite, and a dramatic improvement in her anemia. Within five days she was able to return home from the hospital, and, although she died about three months later as expected, she was able to live quite an active and comfortable life until her death. The critical factor in these admittedly anecdotal recoveries was expectant faith, whether or not objectively justified.

Part of the placebo response seems to involve the meaning of the disorder or the illness to the person. Henry Beecher noticed something important in a study of soldiers wounded on a beachhead in the Pacific during World War II: Only a quarter of the wounded needed medication for their pain. These were injuries which would usually require strong medication if civilians suffered them. Tissue damage was similar and yet the wounded soldiers' need for medication was significantly lower. Something had replaced the effect of the drug.

What?

Beecher's insight was that the *meaning* of the pain for a soldier was significantly different from that experienced by a person severely injured in a car accident. For the soldier the wound was a ticket home, a way to get out of the war. For the rest the accident would mean the loss of work, more hospital bills, the loss of free time at home, and more.

One soldier, because of his expectations and its meaning, might welcome the pain; the other might not. And a consideration of the experiences of different soldiers makes a further interesting point. Those who were *less* badly hurt experienced *more* pain and required more pain medication. These soldiers knew that the less serious wounds meant that they would be patched up and sent back to fight—these people actually felt the pain more and required more pain medication.

The way in which a treatment is given also shapes the likelihood of a placebo response. Researchers Steven Gryll and Martin Katahn investigated the impact of the patient's confidence in his or her therapist. Two groups of patients were given the same placebo pill prior to the injection of a dental anesthetic, but each group received a different message about the likely effects of the pill.

The oversell message went something like this: "This is a recently developed pill that I've found to be very effective in reducing tension, anxiety and sensitivity to pain. It cannot harm you in any way, and it becomes effective almost immediately."

The undersell message: "This is a recently developed pill that reduces anxiety, tension, and sensitivity to pain in some people. Other people receive no benefit from it. I personally have not found it to be very effective. It cannot harm you in any way, and if it is going to have an effect, it becomes effective almost immediately."

There was quite a significant reduction in anxiety and pain perception in the patients receiving the confident, enthusiastic message compared to the other message. The influence of confidence was noted as far back as 1833 when the French physician Armand Trosseau advised: "You should treat as many patients as possible with new drugs while they still have the power to heal."

Although confidence on the part of the physician or healer may be helpful, it is not always necessary. In the final analysis all that seems to matter is what the patient believes, whether that belief is objectively correct or not. Lawrence D. Egbert, an anesthesiologist, recalls the case of a patient undergoing an amputation of her foot for diabetic gangrene.

> She was 85 years old, poor and close to illiterate. She accepted spinal anesthesia. Three surgeons were operating while talking about things of considerable social interest in their personal lives. The surgeons were asked to lower their voices but would not. The patient wondered what was going on and seemed only slightly mollified when I told her a birthday party was being held in the office nearby. The young surgeons simply would not quit their joking and horseplay. Finally, the senior surgeon was pouring an antibiotic wash over the raw stump, and the junior surgeon was citing data to show that this activity was a waste of time, when the third surgeon began a loud and humorous pseudoreligious incantation over the ablutions. The patient jumped and again was confused, wondering what was going on. The surgeons stopped the horseplay. The patient, however, took a completely new attitude about the entire business. She thought it was wonderful. Imagine, how nice it was to have fine young surgeons praying over her foot and she just a poor old lady from the country! She was completely impressed with what a fine hospital we had and how nice we all were, and she went on to make a satisfactory recovery. I have no doubt that her recovery was helped by the spiritual support she thought she was receiving.

The importance of the suggestions given with any treatment is further illustrated by a case described by psychologist Neil Fiore. He describes his own experience when he was treated with chemotherapy for cancer. He suggested that the distress from side effects, such as hair loss, extreme nausea, and vomiting, might be reduced if the treatment were introduced with a positive rather than negative message.

> Physicians, by their attitudes and words, can lead patients to imagine and expect a hopeless situation with much pain. Examples of this approach are, "You will have a lot of pain but we have the drugs to help you," or "Chemotherapy is highly toxic and you will lose your

hair and become nauseated." By the same token, aware physicians can use the patient's suggestible state to calm and to increase the chances for a positive outcome.

They can say, "You will be receiving some very powerful medicine capable of killing rapidly producing cells. Cancer is the most rapidly producing cell, but there are other rapidly producing cells such as hair. And since the medication cannot tell the difference between hair and cancer cells, you may lose some hair temporarily. Fortunately, your normal, healthy cells can recover from the medication and reproduce themselves, but the weak, poorly formed cancer cells cannot."

The positive statement uses the word "medication" instead of "drugs" to emphasize the helpful nature of chemotherapy, and uses "powerful" instead of "toxic" to emphasize the point that this is a strong ally to the body. The loss of hair and other side effects are presented as possible, and not certain, to avoid self-fulfilling prophecies. Most importantly, the statement allows patients to conceptualize the side effects as a sign that their powerful ally is working at killing rapidly producing cells. Without this kind of intervention, patients often conclude that the side effects are proof that they are dying—if not from cancer, from its treatment.

The message given with a treatment can also influence how rapidly it takes effect. In a study of thirty patients undergoing relaxation training to lower blood pressure, half the patients were told their blood pressure would begin to decline immediately following the first training session while the others were instructed that their blood pressure response would be delayed until at least after the third session. Those who expected an immediate response showed a seven times greater reduction (17.0 versus 2.4 millimeters of mercury) in systolic blood pressure when compared with those led to expect a delayed response. The relaxation training was otherwise identical in both cases.

But the effects of these placebo and drug effects are quite complicated. In most cases there exist two factors—a drug which has, or is hoped to have, some real pharmacological effect, and the positive, negative, or neutral effects of the placebo which adds to the drug. These relationships are often difficult to see in normal medical practice, since they always occur together.

But like the placebo operation, specific case histories can sometimes help separate specific physiological effects from placebo effects. In one, a physician gave a patient a new and experimental drug which he hoped would help the patient's severe asthma. The patient reported marked relief in symptoms and improvement on lung function tests.

The doctor was curious. He wondered whether the obvious improvement was due to the new drug or the placebo. So he next treated the patient with a placebo rather than the experimental drug. Sure enough, the patient returned to the doctor and complained once again of his condition, saying that the drug no longer worked. So the good doctor checked with the drug company and requested more of the experimental drug.

The company told him that the "effective" experimental drug was a placebo.

The patient responded in both cases to the *doctor's* differing expectations of the treatment. The doctor communicated to the patient in very subtle ways, perhaps tone of voice, facial expressions, or word choice, whether he thought the treatment would be efficacious or not.

Although we can see these therapeutic effect quite clearly in selected studies, this placebo effect shadows every move of the physician and probably accounts for some of the improvement noted with every medical intervention.

The physical characteristics of the therapy as well as the way it is administered also influence patient expectations and the placebo response. In this instance form seems to matter more than substance; placebo injections are more potent than placebo pills. Placebo capsules are more effective than placebo pills but less effective than injections. Further, small yellow pills seem to work well for depression while large blue pills have a better effect as sedatives. Also, for some as yet undiscovered reason, a very large brown or purple pill or a very small bright red or yellow pill seems to produce better effects than other size or color combinations. In addition, the more bitter-tasting the medicine or difficult and unpleasant the treatment, the more likely a strong placebo effect will be found. Although there are not many studies of placebo surgery except for the one reported earlier, we would guess that it is quite close to the ultimate in placebos.

A recent British study even found that brand names add to the placebo response. Women who regularly suffered from headaches were given aspirin or a placebo in either a familiar and well-known branded packet or an unfamiliar one. Approximately 40 percent of the group receiving the unbranded placebos reported the pain was considerably better. Fifty percent reported relief with branded placebos, 56 percent with unbranded aspirin, and 60 percent with branded aspirin. So while the active ingredient in aspirin was slightly more effective than the sugar pill, the effectiveness was increased by the packaging and the expectation. Do not accept generic placebos!

All of this discussion of the powerful effects of placebos is not to argue for their immediate and liberal use in clinical practice. The ethical issues concerning deception of the patient pose serious barriers to placebo therapy. The real import of the placebo is that it gives testimony to the fact that we have within us certain self-healing mechanisms, intrinsic healing systems, which can be mobilized by appropriate cues which foster a sense of positive expectancy.

The placebo is a tangible symbol that something is being done to help the patient. It evokes a network of strong personal and cultural expectations that the patient will improve. In our society, with its belief in better living through chemistry and worship of technology, what better symbol than a pill? It satisfies our need for something tangible, visible, which can be credited for the improvement.

Norman Cousins observed:

> The placebo is not so much a pill as a process, beginning with the patient's confidence in the doctor and extending through the full functioning of his own immunological system. The process works not because of any magic in the tablets but because the human body is its own best apothecary and because the most successful prescriptions are those that are filled by the body itself.

But in order to know how these prescriptions could possibly be "filled" we need to know a lot about the detailed code of the language of the brain. And how the discoveries of its electrical and chemical nature make it clearer than ever how thoughts and beliefs are an essential part of the brain's operations.

THE PHARMACY WITHIN:
Beliefs, Endorphins, and the Intrinsic
Pain Relief System

*T*here is a long-standing belief that internal substances affect mood, disposition, and even personality. The ancient Greeks believed there were specific body *humors* that determined mood. A characteristically angry person was thought to have an excess of *bile* and a calm one, too much *phlegm;* hence the descriptions "bilious" and "phlegmatic."

Although the particulars of this ancient conceptualization now appear wrong, its basic premise may not be too far off. Minute quantities of chemical transmitter molecules are the ultimate unit of action of the nervous system. Different concentrations of these various neurotransmitters in the brain may well determine temperament, mood, and the function of the intrinsic healing systems of the brain.

Earlier we thought that there were only a very few such chemicals, perhaps three or four. It now appears that there may be hundreds of different chemical messenger molecules and that these neurotransmitters are the "words" which the brain uses to communicate. These transmitters, with names like acetylcholine, norepinephrine, serotonin, dopamine, and endorphin, are involved in excitability, sleep and dreams, hallucinations, pain regulation, mood, thought—in short, these chemicals underlie all brain functions.

If you could actually get inside and see the brain working, you would see millions of miniature explosions going on and off each instant as neurons fired their electrical charges. If you could get inside a neuron itself, you would see scores of chemicals being released, going from cell to cell and back. In the pattern and in the chemical composition of those explosions lie our thoughts as well as the messages sent from the brain to the body.

The brain communicates with and controls the body through this continuous flow of chemical messages: neurotransmitter molecules conveying messages between cells, and neurohormones produced and secreted by the brain carrying messages through the bloodstream to distant target organs. In this sense each nerve cell, and the brain itself, is like an internal pharmacy dispensing a stream of powerful drugs to influence and control moods, thoughts, and bodily functions.

The internal pharmacy has many distinct advantages over the modern corner drugstore, and pharmaceutical companies. First of all, the pharmacopeia of the brain has developed over countless millions of years, a rather long time for research and development. Further, evolutionary experimentation is not limited by the same ethical considerations which complicate research on human subjects. Many organisms were sacrificed by failed drug experiments which did not produced the hoped-for evolutionary advantage. In spite of complaints about the FDA's bureaucracy and the slow pace of introduction of new drugs, these delays pale in the face of the slow, painstaking timeline for the introduction and refinement of the drugs of the internal pharmacy. The evolutionary approach offers millions of years to observe for deleterious side effects and to withdraw from the market drugs which do more harm than good.

The internal pharmacy has also developed drug delivery systems which greatly exceed the sophistication and abilities of our modern medications. Through a network of nerves reaching even the most remote areas of the body, the brain is able to control precisely the amount and timing of the release of drugs in order to maximize specific desired effects and minimize side effects. Even with all our pills, time-release capsules, injections, infusions, aerosols, skin patches, and implants we can only watch as

unintended side effects develop throughout the body while mar-
veling at the precision of brain-directed drugs.

The key to understanding how the brain communicates
through this array of chemical messages lies in the shape of the
chemicals and their receptors. Distributed throughout the body
on the surfaces of cell membranes are hundreds, perhaps thousands, of different types of molecular structures called receptors.
Each type of receptor has a characteristic three-dimensional
shape, and like a lock, can only be opened or activated by a
chemical key with the correct corresponding shape. Thus every
neurotransmitter and hormone molecule has a specific shape
which can fit only specific receptors. This lock-and-key relationship describes how the chemical messages of the body connect
with their target cells. The messenger molecules move through
the bloodstream or across synapses until they fit the receptors
designed for them. Once the receptor is activated, the activity of
the cell is either stimulated or inhibited. Drugs stimulate body
processes because they can mimic naturally existing substances
in the body, simulating their shape, and therefore can fit as keys
to the "locks" within.

An enormous amount of research over the past few years has
begun to uncover the secrets of this neural, chemical, and body
language. In many ways the discovery of the chemical nature of
the brain has further lessened any distinctions between brain and
body, mind and brain. Knowing that the brain is more a pharmacy than a computer focuses our attention on the important role
of the intrinsic healing systems of the brain.

The internal pharmacy dispenses many different types of
drugs, each playing a role in protecting the stability of the organism. Recently, a new class of internally produced substances,
called endorphins, has been discovered and their role in the intrinsic pain relief systems described. The story of the discovery of
these internal pain relievers actually begins with a flower—the
poppy.

Poppy juice—opium—has been used for thousands of years to
attenuate pain and produce pleasure. Morphine, the major active
ingredient of opium, isolated in the early nineteenth century and
later synthesized in the laboratory, remains the drug of choice for
the treatment of severe pain. The fact that the opiates are effective

painkillers is fortunate for humanity, but also curious. Why should a molecule derived from a plant affect the human brain? Most drugs which act on the brain do so by attaching to specific receptors on neurons, like a key in a lock. Thus it seemed likely that morphine and other opiates produced their analgesic effects by binding to a specific receptor site in the brain.

In 1971 Avram Goldstein of Stanford University presented some experimental evidence implying the existence of opiate receptors and suggestions on how to search for them. Four years later Solomon Snyder and Candace Pert, working at Johns Hopkins University, convincingly demonstrated that there must be opiate receptors in the brain. They took advantage of a newly synthesized drug called naloxone. This drug is very similar in structure and shape to morphine but instead of producing pain relief and euphoria, naloxone very effectively and specifically blocks the action (acts as an "antagonist," in the jargon) of morphine and other opiates. Snyder and Pert assumed that naloxone produced its antagonistic effects by tightly binding to the opiate receptor sites, thereby preventing the opiate molecules from occupying the receptors. They exposed brain tissue treated with morphine to radioactivity and found that tissue absorbed less radioactivity when it was also treated with radioactive naloxone. This meant that both the opiates and naloxone were competing for similar receptor sites.

But why on earth should there be a receptor in the brain that is activated by an extract of the opium poppy? This receptor system is found in all vertebrate brains, not just the human. Therefore, it appears to have evolved at about the time the first primitive vertebrates inhabited the seas, long before there was a poppy plant. The obvious answer seemed to be that the body and brain must make their own opiates, and the receptors are there to be acted on by these natural brain opiates.

Several competing groups of scientists around the world raced to find these natural opiates. John Hughes and Hans Kosterlitz of the University of Aberdeen were the first to succeed in 1975. These researchers isolated a substance from the brains of a variety of animals, including rabbits, guinea pigs, rats, and pigs, that possessed pharmacological properties nearly identical to morphine. They named the substance "enkephalin," meaning "in the head." The active ingredient proved to be a mixture of two small peptide molecules.

At first glance these brain "morphines" did not seem to resemble the morphine molecule at all. Peptides are larger molecules constructed of chains of amino acids, which are among the most basic constituents of living cells. Morphine is not a peptide and has a very different chemical structure.

However, when the three-dimensional shape of the morphine molecule is examined, one end of it closely resembles one end of the enkephalin molecule. So what we have been calling the opiate receptors in the brain are, of course, not opiate receptors at all; they are enkephalin receptors, acted on by the naturally occurring brain opioids. Morphine and structurally related synthetic drugs have a shape that fits the opiate receptor.

Indeed, naloxone, the synthetic drug that antagonizes and blocks the effect of opiates, fits the opiate receptors in the brain even better than morphine. This is why it antagonizes the actions of morphine so effectively. It literally knocks the morphine molecule off the receptor and attaches to the receptor. However, its shape is such that although it attaches to the receptor it does not activate it. Naloxone simply attaches and prevents morphine and other opiates from acting on it.

Morphine, opium, heroin, and other opiates, on the other hand, activate the opiate receptors to produce their effects. Since opium was known to produce euphoria, it was thought that the endogenous opiates might also produce pleasurable psychological effects. If naloxone blocked these pleasurable feelings, then it was likely that the endorphins (*endo*genous mor*phines*) were involved. This could not be studied directly.

So, one day in Avram Goldstein's laboratory, the researchers sat around, having been asked the question, "What do you think we can do, in the lab, without much equipment, to stimulate strong pleasure?" It has been reported that the group members all looked at their feet and shuffled around for a while. Finally one young woman made the suggestion, and the experiment was tried. Modesty forbids us from describing it, but the title was "Failure of naloxone to reduce thrills from masturbating to orgasm."

However, some thrills *have* been impaired using naloxone. In a calmer study the research group played its favorite musical passages after the injection of naloxone. They rated passages that normally sent chills up their spine to be less exciting under naloxone, suggesting that the endorphin system has a role in the pleasure derived from music. However, naloxone is more useful than that, as it can vigorously get rid of opiates lodging in the brain.

Among other effects, heroin depresses breathing. A heroin addict who is about to die from a respiratory arrest due to an overdose of heroin will be fully awake and recovered in seconds after an injection of naloxone and will also then immediately exhibit severe withdrawal symptoms. Naloxone displaces the heroin from the brain's opiate receptors and therefore counters the respiratory depression caused by the heroin.

Since the discovery of enkephalins in 1975, a number of other naturally occurring brain opioids have been uncovered, and some are considerably more potent than morphine. One of the peptides, dynorphin, is nearly two hundred times stronger than morphine as a pain reliever. The quest for discovery of new endorphins continues. In early 1986 it was even found that the brain produces traces of morphine. The actions of the brain opioids seem identical to the actions of morphine—they relieve pain and anxiety.

One might think that these substances would prove to be the ideal painkillers, being both potent analgesics and not addictive. After all, they are naturally occurring substances in our bodies. Unfortunately, the endorphins have proven to be just as addicting as morphine and heroin. (Heroin, incidentally, was also originally thought to be nonaddictive and was used to cure morphine addiction!) It seems that any substances that act on the opiate receptors in the brain to relieve pain and induce pleasure are likely to be addicting.

The endorphins *are* powerful analgesics. In 1980, Hiro Oyama in Japan reported the results of the first tests on humans. Fourteen cancer patients with previously intractable pain were given spinal injections of beta-endorphin. All of the patients experienced significant relief from pain, lasting an average of 33.4 hours, and, in one case, for more than three days.

How exactly do the opiates diminish the sensation of pain? British scientists have recently uncovered a possible mechanism. One of the major neurotransmitters involved in the transmission of pain impulses to the brain is a peptide known as "Substance P." In 1977 Leslie Iverson and T. M. Jessell reported that morphine inhibited the release of Substance P. Pretreatment with naloxone blocked morphine's effect on Substance P. As you probably would guess, tests with the endogenous opiates showed exactly the same results as with morphine.

Why do we have opioid substances in our brains? In many circumstances it makes sense that we should have a nervous system which can both transmit and modify pain sensation. Pain signals can prompt recuperation and healing by motivating the organism to withdraw, lessen activity, and rest. However, this response can be counterproductive if there is an immediate need to flee or fight. Therefore, it would be helpful if the organism had some internal mechanism which would dampen pain sensation and permit the organism to ignore physical trauma in order to handle an immediate threat.

Recent research findings support this view. With certain types of stress, the brain appears to trigger the release of endorphins along with ACTH from the pituitary gland. The ACTH is a signal to the adrenal glands to prepare for flight or fight, while the endorphins may help block pain so that the organism can take action without being completely distracted. We know from the way the brain's priority systems are organized that pain stimuli usually get direct access into consciousness and can dominate behavior. The intrinsic pain relief system provides a way to at least temporarily block the pain stimuli and allow appropriate action to be taken.

Consider the numerous accounts of people during battle, accidents, or sporting events who don't even notice the pain from injuries. Could this be due to an activation of our natural capacities for pain suppression? Stress and pain itself appear to be important cues for turning on the intrinsic pain relief system. During the stress of labor it appears that endorphins are released to help the mother and fetus withstand the pain. This was demonstrated in a unique experiment by neurochemist and mother Huda Akil, who allowed her amniotic fluid to be analyzed during the different phases of labor and found that endorphins increased greatly.

At about the same time endorphins were discovered, another dramatic series of studies on pain was taking place. Researchers found that some otherwise intractable pain could be alleviated by electrical stimulation of certain parts of the brain, particularly the brain-stem gray matter surrounding the cerebral ventricles (periaqueductal gray [PAG] and periventricular gray [PVG]).

Cerebrospinal fluid was collected from three patients before, during, and after they underwent PAG stimulation. Concentrations of endorphinlike substances in the fluid increased two to four times as a result of the stimulation. The best results for pain relief came when areas containing the most opiate receptors were stimulated. Repeated stimulation brought increased relief. Microinjections of opiates into these brain areas also produced pain relief, and naloxone was found to block stimulation-produced pain relief, suggesting that endorphins mediate, at least in part, this type of analgesia.

So there exists an intrinsic analgesia system, a natural circuit within the nervous system which acts to relieve pain. The system is complex, involving several pathways; some mediated through the production and release of endorphins, some involving other neurotransmitters and substances. It can be activated by drugs, electrical stimulation, and stress, and even pain itself seems to turn on the system. There is also evidence that acupuncture, an ancient treatment for pain in which needles are inserted into various specific points on the body, may involve an activation of this intrinsic system for pain relief. A recent study suggests that acupuncture analgesia may be mediated by endorphins.

Ten patients suffering from chronic pain were successfully treated for pain with electroacupuncture, a modern variant of acupuncture in which an electrical current is applied to acupuncture points. Following treatment, cerebrospinal fluid concentrations of endorphin rose in all ten. Naloxone has also been shown to block acupuncture analgesia, further supporting a role for endorphins.

Some of the techniques of the folk medicines may well stimulate the internal pharmacy. Might beliefs alone do it?

Although the placebo effect has been known and used for centuries, its mechanism has seemed inexplicable and mysterious until recently. An experiment performed in 1977 by researchers at the University of California at San Francisco suggests that endorphins may mediate at least one aspect of the placebo effect, placebo-induced pain relief.

Almost everybody has heard that morphine is a powerful painkiller. If you are in pain and your doctor gives you a pill or injection of what he says is morphine, you will not be surprised if your pain decreases or vanishes.

However, you might well be surprised to learn that your pain may also lessen if you actually receive an inert substance with no specific pharmacological properties—a placebo. It is a remarkable testimonial to the power of expectations on experience that approximately one-third of patients experience significant relief from pain after receiving placebos.

Jon Levine, Newton Gordon, and Howard Fields at the University of California in San Francisco studied postoperative pain in fifty-one men and women undergoing surgical removal of impacted wisdom teeth. The patients consented to postoperative treatment with either morphine, a placebo, or naloxone (which might increase pain).

After they had their wisdom teeth removed under standard anesthesia, the patients spent several hours in a recovery room, where the experimental drugs were administered and pain was measured. Two hours after anesthesia had begun all patients received a randomly selected injection of either morphine, naloxone, or a placebo. One hour later they received another injection. Neither patients nor researchers knew which substances had been administered until after the experiment. Seventeen patients received a placebo both times, twenty-three patients received a placebo followed by naloxone, and eleven received naloxone followed by a placebo.

Patients receiving a placebo as the first injection were divided into two groups: placebo responders and nonresponders. Responders were defined as those patients who reported less pain one hour after receiving the placebo compared with ratings five minutes before the placebo injection. Nearly 40 percent of the patients were classified as responders by this definition.

When responders received a high dose of naloxone as the second injection, they reported significantly increased levels of pain. When nonresponders received naloxone as the second injection, they reported no changes in pain levels. Pain ratings for responders after naloxone were approximately the same as those for nonresponders. Since naloxone blocks the effects of opiates and endorphins this demonstrated that a major part of placebo analgesia is mediated by the production of endorphins.

In a subsequent series of carefully controlled experiments, Levine and Gordon were able to demonstrate that the potency of the placebo was approximately equivalent to 8 milligrams of morphine. Their elegant experimental design included situations in which the patients were given a placebo openly by someone at the bedside, given a placebo in a hidden manner by a person in an adjacent room, or given a placebo by a preprogrammed infusion pump unbeknownst to anyone.

The preprogrammed machine infusion produced, as expected, no placebo effect. However, they found a significant decrease in pain when the placebo was admininstered openly *or* by the "hidden" infusion from the adjacent room. Surprisingly, when the patients receiving the "hidden" placebo infusion were interviewed after the experiment, they were not able to identify any clues signaling when the "hidden" infusions might have occurred. This suggests that the "hidden" infusion was accompanied by unintentional cues which elicited a placebo response, cues which neither the experimenter nor the patients were consciously aware of. This illustrates how subtle communication can significantly influence therapeutic outcome.

Many other effects apart from pain relief have been observed with placebos, so it is unlikely that endorphins mediate the whole range of responses to placebos. But findings such as those presented here have led many researchers to wonder whether psychological factors such as emotional state, mood, "will to live," and the doctor-patient relationship may not turn out to be as important as drugs in that they promote the synthesis and release of endorphins and other compounds in the brain.

The details of the chemical nature of the brain are just becoming known. We have illustrated here only one of many intrinsic healing systems which are mediated by the internal pharmacy. These physiological links may stimulate a renewed inquiry into the role of emotional and mental factors in preventing disease and restoring health. It could be that the healing rituals of "primitive" societies and folk medicine have real biological effects by helping to stimulate the brain's own healing system. It is likely that additional physiological links will be found with more research on this new view of the brain. At a minimum we should be able to learn how to better coordinate medical therapies with the brain's own efforts to heal itself. And there may be other, more direct ways of igniting these intrinsic healing systems.

CHAPTER SIX

GREAT EXPECTATIONS:
On the Mental Reduction of Warts and Enlargement of Breasts

*I*n the placebo effect, profound physiological changes can be prompted by the suggestion of benefit which accompanies medical treatments. In a sense we exist in a sea of suggestions, symbolic messages which shape beliefs and, in turn, influence our physical well-being. Sometimes these suggestions can be used deliberately, as in hypnosis, to mobilize positive expectancy and alter bodily function in ways that have not been fully appreciated.

Hypnosis isn't a "state" of consciousness, like dreaming. If one hypnotizes a person with the suggestion to behave as if alert, then to all outward signs that person will appear alert. If the person is instructed to relax, then the signs will be as if he were relaxed. Hypnosis is not a unitary or consistent state like dreaming. Hypnotized students are able to alter their skin and body temperature like yogis. Pain thresholds can be raised and memory increased.

Being hypnotized enables a person to access the brain in a way that normal life does not allow. It is often reported that pain thresholds are raised through hypnosis, yet for an understanding of the different systems of the brain and mind this raises a major question: During hypnotic analgesia is the pain completely inaccessible to consciousness, or, rather, is the pain not attended to as usual?

The latter seems the case. In an ingenious hypnotic procedure, Ernest Hilgard of Stanford University elicited two different reports of pain experience. The subjects were hypnotized, given the suggestion that they would not experience pain, and then a pain stimulus was applied. As expected, they verbally reported an absence of pain. However, if they were also given the suggestion that some part of their consciousness might be able at the same time to experience the pain, this "hidden observer" was able to signal by moving a finger that they felt the pain. The hidden observer is an important demonstration that many experiences below consciousness may enter it through hypnosis. This split indicates the large control we possess over consciousness, at least over our criteria for reporting events, although it is necessary to devise such a study to see this control.

Hypnosis can also show how easily our mental shifts can result in bodily changes. Still, even today most of us do not believe in these capacities. Our perspective is often too similar to that of the Royal College of Physicians of England in the 1850s, when the British surgeon Esdaile demonstrated hypnotic anesthesia for amputation of a gangrenous limb. During and after the operation the patient was obviously awake and not in pain, yet the physicians who observed the procedure discounted the "anomalous" information in front of them. In the *Lancet*, a respected British medical journal, it was asserted that "the patient was an imposter who had been trained not to show pain." Another nonplussed observer reported that Esdaile must have hired a "hardened rogue" to undergo the operation for a fee!

Today we have even more remarkable examples, anecdotal as well as experimental, which demonstrate how the body can be altered in profound ways through hypnosis and suggestion.

One of the authors, David Sobel, was plagued with warts as a child. He says:

From the ages of about eight to twelve a nasty collection of warts populated my hands and feet. The warts, usually numbering about a dozen, were painful, unsightly, and recalcitrant. For nearly four years I made pilgrimages to dermatologists. They burned, needled, cut, cauterized, froze and even X-rayed these growths, but to no avail. One wart might be temporarily deterred, but would then regrow the moment there was a lull on the battlefield. I came to respect the tenacity of these accursed growths.

Then a remarkable thing happened. I remember the day vividly. My mother handed me a newspaper clipping with the headline, "Warts Cured by Suggestion." My curiosity was aroused. I read on. The article described some research which suggested that warts could be permanently arrested by hypnosis. I glanced down at the nasty, scaly cutaneous eruptions. Could something as simple as suggestion stand a chance against these formidable opponents? I figured it was worth a try. The only problem was, they didn't tell in the article how the hypnosis was done.

Undeterred, I decided, though by what means I am still not sure, that I must concentrate intensely on the warts while repeating ten times (it had to be exactly ten times) the phrase "Warts go away, warts go away. . . ."

I did this faithfully every day for about four weeks, at the end of which time the warts were but a memory. They had all vanished. From time to time I have had an inkling that one might be attempting to rally, but it has been easily held at bay by a simple recitation of "warts go away" (ten times exactly).

Returning to more formal accounts: Holly, a nine-year-old fourth grader began to develop warts during her first year in grammar school. The growths started on her left hand, but to her considerable dismay subsequently spread. She was unmercifully teased by her schoolmates, and consequently her grades at school declined. At last count she had thirty-one warts on her hands and face. These warts had survived the best conventional medical treatment had to offer, so she agreed to participate in a study of hypnotic treatment of warts.

Holly didn't know much about hypnosis but readily agreed to participate in this novel "kind of game," as it was presented. She took to the hypnosis avidly. She was told under hypnosis to feel a tingling sensation in the warts. After she felt the tingling she was told that the warts would go away in a week or possibly longer. The warts began to disappear after the first session. By the fifth session only five remained, and by three months only two small warts persisted on her left hand.

A coincidence? Perhaps. But "wart stories" such as this are quite common. Everyone seems to have a folk remedy for warts. Rub a cut potato on the wart, paint the wart with food coloring, handle a certain animal, and so on. As varied as these and many other unlikely treatments are they all share in common an intense belief that the treatment will work.

Consider Dr. Bruno Bloch, the famous "wart doctor" of Zurich. He had an enormous reputation for success in curing warts. In his office stood an impressive "wart-killing" machine, with flashing lights, a noisy motor, and "powerful X rays." His patients were instructed to place their affected body parts on the machine and not to remove it until they were told that the warts were dead.

Then the warts were painted with a brightly colored harmless dye and patients were told that they must not be washed or touched until they had disappeared. Indeed, in thirty-one percent of cases studied, Dr. Bloch reported a complete disappearance of all warts after just one treatment. This is much higher than is typically reported for "spontaneous regression"—the routine disappearance of warts in untreated people.

Later controlled studies have shown that warts can sometimes indeed be wished away. A. H. C. Sinclair-Gieben and D. Chalmers reported in 1959 of their success in hypnotic treatment of fourteen patients with intractable generalized warts on both sides of their bodies. The subjects were hypnotized and instructed that the warts on one side of their body would disappear, while the other side would serve as the control. Within several weeks the warts in nine of the patients had regressed significantly but only on the treated side. The untreated side had as many warts as ever except in one subject, whose warts on the untreated side also showed spontaneous disappearance six weeks after the treated side had been cured.

In a later study by a group at Massachusetts General Hospital, nine of seventeen patients treated with hypnosis demonstrated significant wart regression while none of an untreated control group showed any improvement.

So why get excited about the disappearance of a few warts by suggestion? Warts are tumors, benign overgrowths of the skin caused by a virus infection. The virus is ubiquitous, and since not everyone develops warts some type of immune defense must protect the majority of people. The mental wart cures presumably work by either activating the immune system or by altering the blood flow to these growths, or both.

Consider the how elegant is the mind's approach: quick, painless, no side effects and no scars compared to the crude freezing, burning, cutting, and cautery of employed in the modern medical treatment of warts.

Furthermore, think what is involved in the mental cures. The brain must translate such vague suggestions as "warts go away" into detailed battle plans. Chemical messengers are sent to marshal the cells of the immune system in an all-out assault on the virus-induced tumor. Or perhaps small arterioles are selectively constricted, strangling the wart but sparing neighboring healthy skin. A remarkable feat.

And these warts are not vague, functional "psychological" complaints. They are visible, tangible, organic tumors responding to beliefs. Consider how much we could learn from a serious study of wart cures.

Warts are not the only body tissues found to be susceptible to mental control. While warts can be shrunk by suggestion, it appears that breasts can be enlarged. Willard performed a controlled study of thirty-two women between the ages of nineteen and fifty-four. Before treatment an independent observer made careful breast measurements—height, diameter and circumference—of all the women. The women were then treated for twelve weeks. In each weekly session they were given suggestions for deep relaxation and told to imagine warm water flowing over their breasts, to imagine a heat lamp warming the breasts and to feel them pulsating. Tape recordings were made of these suggestions so that the women could practice at home on their own.

Nearly 85 percent of the women were found to have some breast enlargement with 46 percent requiring a larger bra size. Careful measurement revealed an average increase in breast size of one-and-a-third inches in circumference, over one inch horizontally, and two-thirds of an inch vertically. The breast size changes were not correlated with changes in weight or menstrual cycle. These findings are consistent with four other published reports of breast augmentation by suggestion.

The mechanism of breast enlargement by suggestion is not known. It may involve selective dilatation of blood vessels in the breast leading to engorgement or, perhaps, a hormonally triggered proliferation of breast tissue. Again, in either case, the brain must be responsible for mediating this selective tissue growth in response to suggested mental imagery.

Finally, consider the inhibition or triggering of allergic skin reactions by suggestion alone. We all know that certain plants like poison ivy and poison oak can cause a terrible itching, weeping, and blistering of the skin. The skin eruption is an allergic reaction to the oil of the plants and is mediated by the immune system. But who would think that thought alone could either cause a similar skin eruption or inhibit it?

Two Japanese researchers performed an imaginative series of experiments on thirteen high school boys who were known from numerous previous skin eruptions to be highly allergic to a certain plant. Five of the boys were given a hypnotic induction with repeated suggestions of relaxation and drowsiness. The other eight were not given a formal hypnotic induction but were merely given strong suggestions. With their eyes closed all the boys were then told that they were being touched on the arm with the leaves of the poison ivy–type plant. In fact, they were being touched by the leaves of a harmless plant.

All of the thirteen boys demonstrated some degree of dermatitis (including itching, redness, papules, swelling, and blisters) in response only to their *belief* that they were being touched by the poison ivy–like leaves.

Then the experimenters reversed the procedure. This time each boy was told they were being touched by the leaves of a harmless plant when, in fact, they were being stroked on the arm with the poison ivy–type leaves. In this situation when led to believe that the leaves were harmless, eleven of the thirteen boys did not react to the poison leaves with their usual skin eruption. The subjects' thoughts and beliefs were able to turn on or turn off the allergic skin reaction.

Numerous other examples demonstrate the potential for mental influence of physiological states. Redness, swelling, and blistering of the skin can be prompted by suggestion alone. The inflammation resulting from a burn can be minimized. Bleeding following a tooth extraction can be decreased. Studies of those trained in biofeedback, yogis, and other psychophysiological athletes demonstrate that we have greatly underestimated the impact of thoughts on physiology.

Obviously there are limits to the ability to be able to deliberately influence and control bodily functions through mental means. Yet the impact of intangibles like words and symbols, when leveraged through a brain whose major form of exchange is such thoughts, can be powerful. Words can be scalpels. They can generate thoughts, feelings, and beliefs in our brain which can be communicated to the cells of our body and even to the chemicals within cells. Our cells can change their activity to conform to the messages which are continually being received from ourselves and others. We have only begun to explore the potential of this "psychosomatic plasticity."

SMALL WORLDS, SMALL BRAINS:
Making Up Your Mind

A ll this discussion of "the faith that heals," or the importance of the interpretation compared with reality, or belief, the value of words as scalpels, may seem like fairy-tales from a mechanical medical viewpoint. After all, beliefs are so intangible, ethereal, constantly shifting and changing. How could they compare with, let alone influence, the solid stability of the "real world" of organs, tissues and cells? Our experience of the world seems so stable and continuous: rich with color, shapes, thoughts, and ideas. The house we live in is the same from day to day; our friends are the same; the world of colors, lights and sounds goes on; the robins come back every year; the smell of autumn is the same.

But our experience of a stable outside world is a *consistent illusion that the brain creates*. It is an illusion that has been "designed" long before we arrived on earth, for the purpose of biological survival. The illusion begins at the first neuron. Our senses grab only a little of reality; the eye takes in a trillionth of the energy which reaches it, the ear similarly. So, our experience of the world as stable is so because of the way the brain is organized, not because of the way the world is.

Consider the problem which confronted the brain early in evolution. Since the world is constantly changing, the brain is flooded with information. How would it know which of all these changes are important and which are irrelevant? How would it know which changes represent real threats to survival and therefore should be attended to immediately? A strategy emerged in which the brain and nervous system evolved to radically reduce and limit the information transmitted to the brain. From this trickle of sensory information a simplified model of the world is calculated. The brain then monitors the sensory input to scan for information which doesn't fit the model or, based on the model, signals a significant threat to which it must react.

The nervous system organizes information so that a few actions, the appropriate actions, can take place. Much of the intricate network of receptors, ganglia, and analysis cells in the cortex serve to simplify. Senses select only a few meaningful elements from all the stimuli that reach us, organize them into the most likely occurrence, and remember only a small organized sample of what has occurred.

Stability in experience is difficult to come by, and evolved over hundreds of millions of years, beginning with the first nerve cell that experienced and simplified the world.

At each step in the pathway from sensory nerve cell to the brain the world becomes more organized and simplified in the mind. A network of schemata is developed to represent the world so that the external world, so chaotic and changing, becomes stable, simplified, and seemingly coherent in the mind. Instead of thousands of reflecting bits of glass, gray stone, scores of doors opening and closing, several high ceilings, we perceive *one* building. The parts fit together.

Although there is a great richness of sensory information reaching us, nevertheless the information we receive at any one moment is often incomplete. We may catch but a glimpse of our friend's shirt or hear only a word or two of his voice, yet we recognize him. In order to organize the world we often need to go beyond the immediate information we receive.

The simple registration of information reaching us somehow does not "add up" to our living experience of our world. Here, for instance, is a simplified and abbreviated example of sensory information as it is transmitted to the brain: "Increasing 700 NM waves in the right, accompanied by increasing pressure of sound waves of 60 to 80 Hz at 40 degrees to the left." Information in this form does not mean much to us. The message "a bear is coming, and fast, on the left" certainly does.

In order to interpret the meaning from "raw" sensory information, the small brain system uses a basic rule of thumb. In effect it asks: What is the simplest *meaningful* thing that the sensory stimuli can be organized into? Thus, we do not experience a "rectangular expanse of red," but a "red book"; when we hear sounds getting louder we know (or assume) an object is approaching; when an object looks smaller and smaller, this *means* it is moving away from us.

The second step in calculating meaning is interpretation. Consider seeing the bear approaching: First the information from the senses is organized into the perception "bear." But what is the meaning of "a bear" in your presence? What action do you take? Suppose the "bear" suddenly says "Trick or treat!" Now you remember it is Halloween, and the meaning of "bear" becomes quite different than if you had heard a growl!

The prime achievement of the organizing processes of the mind is the stability of experience, as there is stability of the internal worlds. The same object presented in very different aspects is experienced as the same. A cup is seen from several different angles. Even though the actual image is different in each instance, you see the same cup. Changes in the slant of an object cause the retinal image to change, but not your experience of the object.

As someone walks toward you from the horizon, that person's "image" on your retina can increase by more than 100 times, but you do not think the person is actually growing larger and larger before your eyes.

Although the brightness and color of an object vary in different illuminations, they are perceived to be the same. The whiteness of the pages of this book will look about the same to you in sunlight as it does in an unlit room at twilight.

The most impressive thing about the mental organizing processes is how little change we experience even though the sensory information reaching us changes radically. As you walk toward a distant building, the visual image shifts from one of a small dot on the horizon to a large building completely filling your visual field. Yet we perceive the building to be the same size and shape regardless of our vantage point. The main purpose of all the receiving, organizing, and interpreting that goes on in the perceptual processes is to achieve constancy, a stable, constant world.

When we have one, we can operate because we know what is going to happen. As you have been reading this book your breathing has been going on. Though you have not been aware of it, some part of your brain has been at work monitoring your breathing. If it had suddenly changed, let's say stopped, you would have immediately become aware of it so that some sort of action could take place. This stable model of the world is the backdrop against which we look for unexpected changes that might signal danger—the irregular heartbeat, the chest pain. This stable view not only alerts us to danger but gives us some sense of control and predictability in a changing world.

The external world appears stable to us because we see so little of it. But the external world is actually much less stable than is our experience of it; its sights, sounds, and germs are not consistent. The cost of our perceived stability is oversimplification. Our own world seems quite simple and organized to us: People remain the same, ideas remain the same, problems remain the same, diseases remain the same, and life goes on. But this simplicity of the perceived world is actually the result of a great deal of brain processing, simplifying the enormous changes in the outside world so that what is experienced is the absolute minimum, so that we can act quickly.

When we are in a good mood, everything seems right with the world: We see it through rose-colored glasses. When we are in a bad mood, everything—from foreign policy to friendships—is seen in a more negative light. There are thoughts and feelings that get hot in the mind and command us: They may be excitement, extreme emotion, an unexplained happening.

Since we do not really experience much of the outside world, our consciousness and our judgments and actions in truth swing around wildly. When you are angry you tend to see others as angry as well, even if they are not. People hypnotized to feel a certain emotion and then taught something remembered what they had learned better when they were again in that emotional state than in another one. These get on the fast track, and when an event enters consciousness, *all associated ideas* are brought forward as well. The presence of a hot idea—like the death of a

king, a common myth, or a ritual supposed to excite and heal—
heats up the rest of the mind and calls information and systems
of the brain into readiness. The arrival of the doctor, the recitation
of a prayer, or the swallowing of a pill can all trigger powerful
associated emotional reactions with profound physiological effects.

In a well-known study on the effect of interpretation on emotion, S. Schacter and J. Singer injected epinephrine, an activating
drug, into a group of unsuspecting students, who were told it
was a new vitamin. Half of the students were then placed in a
room with a euphoric person (a confederate of the experimenters)
who tossed paper airplanes and used the wastebasket to shoot
baskets with wads of paper. These students later reported feeling
euphoric. The other half of the students were confronted by an
insulting and irritated person. They later reported being angry.
So euphoria or anger can be produced by how we interpret a
situation, not only the situation itself.

This particular experiment has had many critics who find that
it is difficult to repeat. Also, many theorists have pointed out that
most often we *do* know what is happening to us: Our senses and
our emotions are well designed to automatically interpret actions
in the world.

Many academic researchers have overemphasized the importance of interpretations, but they often affect us strongly. West-
erners see shrimp, for instance, as a delicious, succulent meal,
while Middle Easterners often look upon it as vermin, much as
we might view a New Guinea meal of squiggling grubs.

Careful research has found that our interpretation of what we
are seeing can literally change physiology. In one study at Richard Lazarus' laboratory at the University of California, Berkeley,
the ubiquitous undergraduate students were made to watch what
was called a very "arousing film." The film was of a ceremony
that an aboriginal tribe used to mark manhood. The rituals included the subincision of the penis with a knife. Most people
found these scenes less than delightful, and, as in the words of
the trade, "negatively arousing."

Arousal of the autonomic nervous system was measured by the
skin resistance (the galvanic skin response) and was charted continuously during the viewing. One group was shown the film
silently. A second group heard a narration that emphasized the
cruelty of the ritual. Two other groups heard narrations that min-

imized the cruelty by denying or intellectualizing it. Arousal increased among those who heard the narration that emphasized the cruelty, while arousal decreased among those who heard the narrations that minimized it.

Growing up, most children have to learn to identify the many changes that go on within them: tiredness, lack of food, frustration, anger. They often misinterpret the signals from their bodies. They may fly into a rage every evening at ten o'clock, and decide they hate their parents, when they are just physically exhausted.

One way to test the theory is to offer false feedback on the internal state itself. If emotional experiences depend in some way on the interpretation of the inner state, then false information should also have an effect on experience. In one study men were shown photographs of nude women while listening to their own heartbeat. What each actually heard, however, was not his own heart beating, but a recording. One group heard a recording in which the heartbeat increased when five of the ten slides were shown. A second group heard "their" heartbeat decrease at these five slides. Later, when asked to rate the attractiveness of the nudes, the group whose heartbeat increased rated the women in the five slides as more attractive; the ones whose heartbeat decreased found the other five more appealing. The false feedback effect is not restricted to men looking at nudes. In another experiment, women were shown slides of people who had experienced violent death. Those who "heard" their heart rate increase in reaction to the slides rated them as significantly more unpleasant and discomforting than those who had not been misinformed.

For instance, many people find that exercise with a partner of the opposite sex is very sexy. Why? In one study people of opposite sexes were asked to exercise together. Later they rated their partners as desirable. The activation resulting from exercise diminishes with time; soon after exercise one no longer *feels* activated; however, measures of autonomic activation, such as blood pressure, are still elevated. If people are shown erotic stimuli during this phase, they report more sexual arousal than when they have fully recovered from the exercise. The unexplained activation is interpreted, again, as sexual excitement. So activation, especially in contrived or ambiguous situations, is subject to interpretation which has practical value for the cad. Many seducers attempt such a hopeful confusion of increases in heart rate. They may involve daring exploits, some deliberate arousing, or risk. Why otherwise would horror movies, roller coasters, or driving absurdly fast be such common teenage pastimes on dates?

Our representation of reality, our beliefs and our feelings about the world are what we act upon, not the world itself. Having a good explanatory model of the world when an unexpected event happens is important to maintaining internal stability—otherwise we don't know whether to panic and run or to ignore a loud noise. Most cultures and most systems of medicine have maintained a set of beliefs about the physical and even spirit world, myths that people live by. A thunderstorm is less cause for alarm if it is immediately interpreted as one of the specific gods growling; a sudden tragedy is explainable if the gods are angry.

The results of all these assumptions about the world, the incessant simplification, interpretation, and effort within the brain are to organize events in a coherent manner so that they can be operated upon or controlled.

And we try to do this at every instance. There is much current research on how people respond to what are called "discontinuities." These are upsets to stability—an insult to one's integrity, a sudden and unexplained noise, internal upsets that are unexplained, a change in one's job or one's life, drought, plague, epidemics, the death of the king, and the like.

What we do when confronted with these sharp changes is to understand what is happening to us and in some cases try to explain them. Consider the situation many people experience when they are getting sick from a flu. They may spend hours, even days feeling badly about their life, their job, their marriage, their energy level, their competence. They may berate themselves and even decide to divorce or quit their job. Then it dawns on them: The hotness, the sweating, and the listlessness were not caused by dissatisfaction with their lives, but by the flu. The complaints about marriage, job, and finances magically disappear once "I'm sick" is registered as the explanation.

We tend to create stories to explain to ourselves and others what is happening inside our bodies as well as without. David Sobel relates:

> I once saw a patient who was suffering from severe hyperthyroidism. His body was responding to the excessive output of thyroid hormone, which whipped his metabolism almost into a frenzy. He had

the classic symptoms of hyperthyroidism: nervousness, palpitations, weight loss, heat intolerance, and so on. But for each symptom he had constructed an explanation. He was nervous because of insecurity about his job. His heart beat rapidly because he often thought about his girlfriend. He had lost weight because he was "eating on the run." He always felt hot because they kept the thermostat too high at his office; and so on.

We are not always right about our interpretations, especially in the modern world, where some of the dangers *are* unprecedented. Psychologists Nelkin and Brown studied workers in plants producing neurotoxic chemicals. For years, the workers complained of fatigue, memory loss, comprehension difficulties, and more. Motivation was lowered, and there were reports of marital discord. But it was the chemicals in the plants causing the reactions, reactions that were explained using the most logical information available to the workers.

Obviously attending to a significant instability has important consequences: The situation may be a novel and real danger. But most often it is something which must be explained and accounted for so that future actions can be planned and the threats in the future reduced.

So we have a built-in bias, it seems, to try to search out explanations for those unusual events. Characteristically we try to make the unfamiliar events familiar, make them seem less like a destabilizing force in our lives. And so we search out logical explanations: The king's death means that the crop-planting cycle was wrong; a tumor means that I am behaving badly; this rumbling in my stomach means that the medicine must indeed be powerful.

But why have all societies evolved these extravagant beliefs and mythologies about the world? Beliefs developed to patch over the gaps between the limited nature of the information that gets inside our brains and the complexity of the world. Our brain is one containing only a few abilities, each one touching small pieces of the world lightly, just enough to get by.

Since we have such a limited system, there are obviously many events which do not fit. Instability in the outside social world is responded to in the body, and any discontinuity in experience causes an immediate reaction: The brain is designed to notice changes.

In order to help us maintain a stable view of the world and our place in it we need a set of simple and consistent beliefs to tell us what to do. Otherwise we'd go crazy with all the instability. The world presents constant challenges and it is often ambiguous, so it is left to the brain to compute a workable reality—a small world —in which the person can operate. But this simplicity, though it brings a kind of stability, also has its cost.

The normal strategies of the mind's operating system—simplification, exclusion of information—make us continually overreact from the little information we finally do select and allow to enter consciousness. When the news reports a murder in a distant city, we tend to think of the world as a more murderous place. When someone famous comes down with breast cancer, it becomes a national concern. When you are frustrated in traffic, you can become frustrated about the progress at work or the state of your marriage as well.

The contents of the mind at any moment are automatically overemphasized no matter how they get there: be it by accident, by direct manipulation, or information remaining in memory. The resident contents cause us to think differently, act differently, and function differently. When people are made happy by hypnosis in psychological experiments or by finding money (either in experiments or in life) or by falling in love, their ideas change, often unknown to themselves. Their opinions about the economy, about the risk of nuclear war, and about their government's performance are all instantly, automatically affected by their mood. They search out different information, make decisions differently. And they are unaware of it.

Just as your spouse, if he or she is annoyed at something on the news, is unlikely at that moment to give you a big kiss, so we all respond to the same information differently depending upon which part of the mind is active at that moment.

Consider this from a different person's "point of view" (the different contents of the speaker's mind). When one person says a glass is "half empty" and another says it is "half full," it is not just a cliché, but a description of how people search their environment differently. One person is looking at what is gone, the empty space; the other is looking at what is left, the liquid.

And consider this classic demonstration: A group of people looked quickly at a set of playing cards and were asked how many aces of spades there were. They all gave a low answer. But for this experiment a few of the aces of spades had been printed in red, and were not registered as such by the viewers. Obviously we search out our world in a simple way, looking only at a few markers to signpost internal experiences. Here our normal "playing card beliefs" direct us to look for black spades only.

In another study, people waiting at a copying machine were asked this question: "Excuse me, may I use the machine for a moment?" Most people refused, suggesting that the person wait his turn in line. But then this variation was tried: "Excuse me, may I use the machine for a moment so that I can make some copies?"

A greater number of people agreed! Our affairs with reality are very selective; we are only looking for what we want at any moment. It is as if we were waiting only for a "reason slot" to become filled in order to act, a slot which is searched only for whether it is filled, not what it means. Why would anyone want to use a copy machine for anything else?

Suppose your doctor told you this after a biopsy: "The chance that you will survive the next six months is only half." And compare it with: "There is a fifty percent chance you will live more than six months." It is not just that the same information is being presented differently in these two very different descriptions. The fragile nature of our beliefs has a great influence on how we may think, how we may react, and what we do.

The shift in perception from the information given in "fifty percent will die" versus "fifty percent will live" is not trivial and could even be a matter of life or death. Hearing about a fifty percent chance of dying may immediately call up the many details one has to take care of before death: the undertaker, the will, the loss of family, of friends and of support for one's children, a loss of the ongoing social connection. A fifty percent chance of living may well call up hopes and ideas for the future, for plans, for projects to be started, and the like. There is literally a shift of mind caused by the information in these different descriptions, a shift far beyond what we might have ordinarily expected. In fact, as we shall see, our own beliefs about our health are quite important.

A sudden pain in the gut might be frightening and might scare one to death, but it might either be hunger pangs or one of the gods sending a message. It is achieving an instant explanation that may allow a person, for instance, to shift less into the emergency reaction to a perceived instability in the world, less into panic and other reactions that may well damage him more than the threat itself. In many ways our simplifying ideas allow us to remain stable in the face of many threats and upsets.

Beliefs control a far greater portion of the mind and the body than we might think, just as the rudder on a two-hundred-thousand-ton supertanker may weigh about one ton, but its setting determines the direction of the whole. With such a mental system composed of a small set of assumptions to cover a wide range of occurrences, it is easy to see that changes in these assumptions will activate different parts of the brain for readiness to act, and thus change the way the body can work. A belief can change the way we see distance, the way we operate, and the way we ready our body for action. That means or at least implies that small changes in the system can make large changes possible, because we live within a very restricted range of information.

What the brain, especially the conscious part, does is first simplify and select information from the outside world. Then it has to know what is going on inside. Then it decides which system to use and plans actions. At any moment the content of consciousness is what we are prepared to act on next: a sudden movement over there, hunger, an idea about our next move, avoiding the stone in front of us, cutting the bread.

Our view of the world is hardly stable in reality. There are various "fast paths" into consciousness: Emergencies, sudden noises, and internal upsets like a toothache have immediate access. Strong emotions, unexpected or very recent events, and striking or vivid occurrences get in unbidden, and once in consciousness can have great effects. Describing this, the thirteenth-century Persian poet Jalāl al-Dīn Rūmi wrote: "What bread looks like depends upon whether you are hungry or not." And thus what is "on our mind," a sudden movement, a belief about a medication or therapy, can have profound consequences. Changing beliefs shifts the mind, so that we may be in essence another person when our beliefs change—we shift the system of the brain which is now operating.

Every system of medicine, whether ancient or modern, works through our beliefs. In addition to whatever direct, specific physiological effect a therapy may have, there is always the symbolic reality and impact of the intervention. All systems of medicine organize the complex worlds of health and illness in terms of explanatory models.

These models simplify the world and help make it seem more coherent and manageable. Even the act of classifying a disease, giving it a name, whether it is called an excess of the fire element in Chinese medicine, an enchantment by Coyote in Navaho medicine, or hyperthyroidism in Western biomedicine, can be therapeutic. The name and explanation domesticates and makes known a wild, frightening phenomenon which threatens personal stability. By transforming the unknown into something known, named, and explained, alarm reactions in the brain can be quieted. Therapies, whether acupuncture, sand paintings, or pills, all have a symbolic value in addition to whatever direct specific effect they may have.

Among other things a sick individual feels isolated, cut off from others by a wall of symptoms and often by fears of contagion. The therapeutic act, no matter what the culture, no matter what the content, serves to reconnect people to others. The diagnosis or explanation of the disease reinforces the patient's connection to the larger social order and social values, which help organize and stabilize the world.

"No Man Is an Island"

CHAPTER EIGHT

PEOPLE NEED PEOPLE

John Anderson, after 37 years of marriage, finds himself alone. His wife died recently from breast cancer. Three months after her death, Mr. A. suffers a fatal heart attack.

Sally Biedermeyer is 26 years old and suffers from asthma which she usually keeps under good control. She recently separated from her husband and has started a new job. She has had three visits to the emergency room for asthmatic attacks in the past two months.

Masa Yamamoto is a 55-year-old electronics worker who left Japan 10 years ago and has since lived in San Francisco. Over the past few months he has been experiencing chest pains and has been diagnosed as having coronary artery disease.

Betsy Larsen has just had a miscarriage. The course of her pregnancy had been complicated by the death of her father with whom she had been very close.

All these people suffered a loss or an extreme disruption in their relationships with family and friends. All have subsequently been more vulnerable to health problems of one sort or another. We all know people who have gotten ill subsequent to the loss of a loved one or after moving to a new city or country and leaving behind friends and family. A coincidence?

Perhaps, but a pattern of susceptibility to disease is apparent in those with disrupted or weakened social ties. People who are single, separated, divorced, or widowed are two or three times more likely to die than their married peers. They also wind up in the hospital for mental disorders five to ten times as frequently. Whether we look at heart disease, cancer, depression, tuberculosis, arthritis, or problems during pregnancy, the occurrence of disease is higher in those with weakened social connectedness.

Most physicians tend to view health and disease as a problem of an individual organism, analyzing each body as though it were entirely separate and discrete. But diseases neither start nor stop at the boundaries of one skin. When an individual is sick, the disorder, whether infectious or not, may spread. Work and personal life become disrupted. Personal relationships may be strained, sometimes to the point of dissolution.

What may begin as a dysfunctioning organ may result in the distress and disease of others. Further, evidence is mounting that health and resistance to all diseases can be influenced by social connectedness.

After all, social forces affect us all the time, just as our interpretations do. They affect us as a current moves all fish in a school, although none of them, looking only at the individual fish next to them, perceive it. And individual physiology does not really stop at the skin boundaries, anyway, nor does our consciousness. Try this: Feel where the pencil you write with touches the page. Note that you do not feel your hands at the point where they grip the tube, but you feel the point of the pencil itself as it moves along the page, a point for which you obviously have no receptors.

But like fish in water, we don't see the unseen hand of others in society. Other people constantly affect our thoughts and our lives, not only directly, but in the way we think and act. Why does a mile runner need pacing to break the record? He needs it because he will run faster with another person around. Bicyclists set records only in competition with others; even little children reel in their fishing lines faster in groups than alone. We need others to know how intelligent we are, what to wear, whether we are good-looking, how to think, act, and feel.

And social factors influence whether a person gets sick in the first place, whether the person seeks care for the sickness, whether the person follows the medical advice, and whether the person recovers. Ignoring the social dimension of health and disease limits drastically the effectiveness of medicine.

In 1897 the French sociologist Émile Durkheim published his classic study of suicide. He commented that while suicide was the most individualistic act one could imagine, the occurrence of suicide followed a pattern understandable only from a social perspective. Suicide rates were higher for Protestants than for Catholics, higher for the unmarried than for the married, higher for soldiers than for civilians, higher in times of both booming prosperity and recession than in times of economic stability.

While individuals may have had different reasons for committing suicide (e.g., financial problems, illness, problems with personal relationships), the suicide rates remained relatively constant over time within each group, whether they were Catholics, Protestants, married or not, even though the individual group members of course changed. Durkheim initially considered factors that were purely cultural, such as the attitude of the groups toward suicide. But he rejected that idea. For instance, Catholics view suicide more negatively than Jews do, but Catholics have a higher rate of suicide. Durkheim reasoned that there must be something in the social organization of the different groups which either predisposed the individuals to suicide or prevented them from killing themselves.

Not only did Durkheim identify that the nature of one's social organization can influence individuals' lives, but he also correctly assessed the *way* the group affects the individual. He maintained that the critical factor in determining suicide was the degree of *social cohesion*—in our terms the stability of the social organization.

Those who were more connected to their own social group were less likely to consider committing suicide, and those social groups that emphasized a strong community also had lower suicide rates. This provided some of the first scientific evidence that an individual's actions, related to his very survival, are influenced to a significant degree by the ways people relate to the others around them.

And there has followed a great deal of new evidence on the relationship of social connections, social disruption, and social disorganization to susceptibility to disease. In a study done in 1972 that confirmed Durkheim, the sociologists Bock and Webber found that widows who had relatives living nearby or who belonged to one or more organizations were less likely to commit suicide than widows who had neither kind of connection.

Another study considered the health problems of the residents of more than one hundred counties in North Carolina. Black males of all ages who lived in a socially disorganized setting had significantly higher death rates from stroke and had higher blood pressure. "Social disorganization" in this case was characterized by family instability, many illegitimate children, single-parent families, separations, and divorces. The increased death rates persisted even when differences in economic status were controlled, supporting the idea that social instability *itself* predisposes people to disease.

Rapid or dramatic changes in one's social world, such as moving to a new neighborhood, city, or country can occasion the subsequent onset of a wide variety of physical and emotional disorders. Even changes in the economy are reflected in the overall incidence of disease. While slow, steady economic growth is clearly associated with lower mortality and longer life, rapid changes in the economy (whether up or down) often result in increased illness.

Recessions which result in unemployment and loss of social status are generally followed by increases in death rates from nearly all causes. Each time the unemployment rate increases by one percentage point, 4 percent more people commit suicide, 5.7 percent more commit murder, and nearly 2 percent more die of cirrhosis of the liver or cardiovascular disease. Some of these responses to economic decline occur rapidly with the onset of the recession while others begin to appear after one to two years.

But it is not just a decline in a life situation, like being let go on the job, that seems to affect health; it is the change in life. Rapid economic *growth,* as well as depression, seems to contribute to mortality. Following a recession, the period of recovery and accelerated economic growth can present special stresses for certain groups of people. Workers who were displaced during the recession face retraining and reentry into the job market during the recovery period.

Further, those who were most vulnerable due to poverty, old age, or sickness during the recession face the added stress of watching others benefit from the economic expansion, not them. Therefore, the result of either recession or rapid economic growth can be more illness in vulnerable social groups.

Social factors not only contribute to disease but can also offer protection. A study by Lisa Berkman and S. Leonard Syme lends credence to the power of social relationships in increasing resistance to disease. In the study, seven thousand residents of Alameda County in California were surveyed and then observed over a nine-year period in an attempt to identify the factors which protect people from illness and death. Many of the questions were standard: smoking, physical exercise, eating habits, history of disease, and the like.

Several questions on the survey, however, dealt with how well people were connected with others. People were asked whether they were married, the number of close friends and relatives they had, and how often they were in contact with these people; they were asked about membership in church and other community organizations. The people ranged from those who were relatively isolated to those very extensively involved with others.

There was a surprising relationship. Those who were single, widowed, or divorced, those with few close friends or relatives, and those who tended not to join or participate in community organizations died at a rate two to five times greater than those with more extensive social ties. These striking differences were true for men as well as women, for old as well as young, for rich as well as poor, and for people of all races and ethnic backgrounds.

Why should this be true? At first glance, one might suppose that at the beginning of the study people who were already sick might report weaker social ties and less community involvement because they were already sick. However, if that were true, the death rates of the isolated people should have been high in the first year or two of the study. But they were not. The people with weak social ties had a higher death rate all through the nine-year follow-up period. Further, these people were asked about their health and illness during the initial interview, and those more isolated did not report any more illness than others.

Further, a subsequent study in Tecumseh, Michigan, which included a medical evaluation at the outset of the study, did not show differences in medical problems which would account for the higher death rates in the socially isolated people.

One might also try to explain the differences on the basis of better health habits on the part of the people with social connections. Could the differences in health be accounted for because people with friends smoked less, exercised more, weighed less, or went to the doctor more for checkups? The social support findings, however, were found to be independent of other traditional risk factors such as smoking, alcohol consumption, exercise, and obesity, as well as the use of preventive health services and reports of life satisfaction. The relationship persisted. The more social connectedness, the lower the death rates.

Another important finding was that the death rates for people who were not stable and well integrated socially were higher for all types of disease, including heart disease, cancer, infections, and accidents. This suggests that social isolation and disconnection somehow increase susceptibility to disease in general. The specific type of disease the person gets depends on the presence of other factors such as genetic predisposition, exposure to carcinogens such as cigarette smoke, diet, lack of exercise, stress, etc.

Such findings suggest a more promising approach to preventive medicine. Instead of studying heart disease, cancer, arthritis, and all the other diseases one by one, we may be able to affect the occurrence of all of them by understanding how social support increases overall resistance to disease. And we may be able to understand some of the underlying psychophysiological mechanisms that affect all disease.

To be sure, social support is only one of many factors which contribute to disease resistance. Genetic predispositions, nutrition, air and water quality, and physical activity may also influence disease susceptibility. Also, some people who are well loved, with a surfeit of friends, do of course become ill and die prematurely, while other isolated people live long, healthy lives. But on the average, there remains a great advantage for those people who have strong, stable connections to others around them.

A vivid example of the importance of social connectedness to health can be seen in a comparison of people living in Japan and in the United States. Both countries are highly industrialized, urbanized, polluted, and exhibit a fast pace of life. Yet Japan has the highest life expectancy in the world and one of the lowest rates of heart disease, only one-fifth the rate in the United States. But this low rate of heart disease seems to hold only for the Japanese who live in Japan. Those Japanese who migrate to Hawaii or California have much higher heart disease rates than Japanese remaining in Japan.

How can we explain these different death rates?

The study of migrants from Japan does not support an explanation based on diet or any simple behavior. When Japanese move to California, those who adopt Western ways show rates of heart disease and other diseases similar to their American neighbors. And there is a gradient—Japanese migrants to Hawaii have a heart disease rate intermediate between those who stayed in Japan and those who moved to California. It seems the farther the migrants got from Japan (or the closer to California), the higher the disease rates.

What is it about America, or at least California, that causes the problem?

Epidemiologists Michael Marmot and S. Leonard Syme identified a subgroup of Japanese migrants to California who had very low rates of heart disease, rates similar to those of their countrymen who remained in Japan. Was it the difference in their diets, an effect on the heart from the higher fat content of the Western diet of cheeseburgers, milkshakes, and fries? Apparently not. The traditional Japanese diet is an extremely high-fat one. All that tempura and raw fish contains lots of fat.

And, comparing people at every level of blood cholesterol, the study showed that the Japanese migrants who maintained strong links to the traditional community had less heart disease. In spite of eating Western foods, having high serum cholesterol, smoking cigarettes, and having high blood pressure, those Japanese with close ties to the traditional Japanese community had low rates of heart disease, a rate only one-fifth as high as those Japanese who adopted a Western pattern of social relationships. These differences in heart disease mortality among Japanese living in different environments cannot be accounted for by differences in diet, cholesterol, smoking or blood pressure level, and consequently has been very hard to explain.

Marmot and Syme noticed that members of the group with very low heart disease rates lived a traditional Japanese life. As children, they had lived in Japanese neighborhoods and had attended Japanese-language schools. As adults their friends were Japanese and they identified with the Japanese community, they visited Japanese doctors, they most often attended Japanese cultural events and Japanese political and social gatherings.

But what does having "close ties to the Japanese community" mean for health? For these people such strong social ties may have prevented a disruption in their social world and their sense of social organization. Like a strong belief system, close ties to others can stabilize a person's view of himself and the world around him. In spite of the numerous inevitable changes, challenges, and disruptions occasioned by migration to a new land, those migrants who retained traditional life-styles remained relatively immune. They maintained a stable view of the world and were able to rely on friends for help and support, thus avoiding the panic, indecision, instability, and illness which often accompany major changes in geographic and cultural circumstances.

Perhaps the more organized, more stable, but even more rigid nature of the Japanese culture, compared with the American one, may also have affected the heart disease rate. Although it is difficult to be precise about this, Japanese society emphasizes social stability and strong social ties more than the American does. In Japan, as many unsuccessful Western businessmen have found, to be autonomous and to stand alone like a rugged cowboy is seen as devious, even pathological. It is the norm in Japan to have lifelong friends, to join and to remain with the same company for a lifetime.

In most of these large companies, there are homes, health care centers, food purchasing plans, social clubs, and a prescribed group of friends. A Japanese man from the Toyota company rarely would go out with competitors from Mitsubishi. The companies are their tribes within the nation. Having a stable place in the world seems fundamental to our nature, and Japanese society speaks to this perhaps more than other societies do.

But it is not only one particular society which protects the heart. Similar results have been found with those Irish who moved to America, who have their own variety of social cohesion, although one less structured than the Japanese. Those who remained in Ireland had lower rates of heart attacks than those who emigrated.

Social support appears to offer a stability which protects people in times of transition and stress. Losing one's job, particularly when it is unanticipated, is understandably stressful and is associated with the development of subsequent illness. But not everyone gets ill when a plant closes or when there is a recession or when a company folds.

The closing of two auto plants in Michigan left hundreds of men without jobs and provided an opportunity to study the protective effects of social support. Susan Gore studied 110 men and found that those who perceived strong support from spouses, relatives, and friends as well as the opportunity to engage in social activities were less likely to have mental and physical health problems. In addition, the men with higher perceived social support were able to adapt to this stressful life challenge with lower cholesterol levels than their less supported counterparts.

Social support also seems to enhance coping with other significant life changes such as pregnancy. K. B. Nuckolls surveyed 170 pregnant women and determined their "psychosocial assets," which relate in part to the amount of support these women perceived themselves as receiving from their families and friends. Ninety-one percent of the complications during pregnancy such as threatened miscarriages and stillbirths occurred in the women experiencing many stressful life events and with low perceived social support. The rate of complications was three times higher in the low support group compared to the women with high levels of perceived support. The perception of good emotional support from families appeared to buffer the effects of the stress, and the course of pregnancy was not adversely affected. Similarly, G. W. Brown and his colleagues found that having an intimate and confiding relationship with a husband or boyfriend reduced the likelihood of depressive symptoms developing in women facing life stresses.

Social support comes in many forms: intimate relationships with friends and family, casual contacts in the community, memberships in religious and other community organizations, work relationships with bosses, employees, and coworkers.

These relationships may help us in very different ways. We can obtain emotional support including reassurance, empathy, and someone to rely on and to confide in, as well as the feeling that we are loved and cared about. We can be encouraged by others to adopt healthier behaviors: to stop smoking, eat regularly, exercise, take prescribed medications, or seek medical care. Friends can provide an invaluable source of information on how to do things, find a job, or locate services. Social support can be a source of money, goods, or services.

Given the complexity of the phenomenon of social support and the relative infancy of research in this area, it is too early to be able to specify the exact mechanisms by which support enhances health. We also need to learn more about which type of support works best in what situation.

For example, in a study of the degree of atherosclerosis of the coronary arteries, Teresa Seeman found that a lesser degree disease was *not* associated with the number of friends or contacts or degree of intimacy. Instead people who felt they had someone they could turn to for help, money, or support were the ones with less coronary artery disease.

We need to understand how social support gets into the body, how our friends communicate with our immune systems, how caring for and being cared for changes our hearts. But part of it seems to involve shifting our attention outside ourselves to the larger group.

This shift can occur because of our association with people,

pets, or even plants. Consider for a moment the strong and enduring relationships people cultivate with pets. And yet classic
medical dogma paints a pretty sad picture for pet owners. You
can be bitten, scratched, or clawed. You can get rabies or ring-
worm or even, from parrots, a rare lung disease. Nevertheless,
people persist in owning pets. Over one-half of American homes
have one or more pets.

There is good news on the health front for pet owners. A study
of heart attack victims one year after the attack revealed that pet
owners had one-fifth the death rate when compared with the
petless. And it didn't seem to matter what kind of pet the person
owned. Since most people don't walk their pet fish or lizards as
they do their dogs, increased physical exercise could hardly account for these striking differences. It may have something to do
with the sense of responsibility experienced by pet owners. They
may have an added incentive to survive in order to continue to
care for their animal companions, who depend upon them. It is
also possible that people who own pets have a different type of
personality which protects them more than the interaction with
the pet itself. Still other studies suggest that interaction with pets
may have a salutary effect: Talking to or petting animals or even
watching fish in a tank lowers blood pressure.

The sense of connectedness and responsibility, whether it be
to people, pets, or plants seems to draw us out of ourselves and
link us to the larger world. The predisposition to communicate
with others, to bond, appears to be vital to our health. It is also
deeply rooted in human evolution.

CHAPTER NINE

FROM THE INDIVIDUAL
TO THE SOCIAL BODY

*I*n addition to performing its myriad of tasks to maintain the internal stability and function of the bodily organs, the human brain seems notably attuned to the social environment. The brain appears prepared to register and respond to changes in the social world, from national tragedies to personal losses. At the same time, the brain seems primed to try to form and maintain stable social relationships, whether to spouses, friends, companies, societies, or even pets.

To understand why human health depends so much upon social stability, it is necessary to first appreciate how the brain evolved and the different forces which shaped its development. This involves examining why we have the kind of infancy and family unit we do and why we have the kind of dependence on others unlike any species.

Human beings possess a network of combined evolutionary changes—from upright posture to a thickened pelvis, from concealed ovulation to sexual pleasure, from tool use to division of labor—which contribute to the survival value of the human "social body." Social groups favor survival in many practical ways: sharing in the protection and bringing up of offspring, cooperation in hunting and gathering, collaborating in defense against predators.

"Society" is often thought of as a separate, somehow incorporeal system, existing apart from the hearts and minds of real bodies. It is studied coldly in sociology treatises almost as if it had its own rules and its own realities. It has been said that to a Marxist you are born only when you apply for a job; to a Jewish mother life begins only when her son graduates from medical school; and for other theorists the world of nations, cultures, and states takes on a life of its own. But to us, human society is a group of biological organisms and is a biological organism in its own right.

The brain is the controller of those organisms; the translator of several simultaneous worlds, the internal molecules, the organs, the individual, the world of what other people are doing, and more. The brain has separate and independent "modular systems," which are specialized to maintain cellular, organ, individual, and perhaps group health. Our evolution has probably selected each of these systems separately for survival.

There are many ways, hackneyed and not, to distinguish human life from that of other animals. We call this the "human beings are the only animal with drapes, the mammal who created car washes, the primate with the needlepoint pattern books, the only organism who has televised contests of dressage" argument. The argument usually asserts that some individual high-level mental function, like creativity, music, a particular development of written language, or the technical abilities stemming from tool use is central to the human spirit and species. In another version, this is the brain-as-a-thought-machine argument.

But there *is* something rather more basically different about us as compared with other species, something which has come to lodge within a part of the human brain. Nesting separate from the rest of it, it includes a complex of new talents involving language, symbol making, and communication which evolved during the long period of human evolution.

It is in part our ability to communicate in symbols, to coordinate with others, relate to them, form flexible and changeable group associations for planting, for hunting, for marriage, for family, for building, for complex tool making, and more that enabled the human species to dominate life on earth. After all, while language and symbolic activity are quite special abilities, there is no sense in having the ability to speak or to write without being able to tell someone what to do! The emergence of the modern human as an important, even dominant species on earth was in large part based upon cooperative efforts in which organized groups could accomplish what no individual could—so cities were built, land was farmed, and industry and technology were created, really, out of nothing. An important part of the specialization of the human brain is to connect individuals together into a larger group, a society, one in which their own chances to survive are improved as are their chances to pass on their genes.

We are social animals, and together form, in a sense, a larger "social body." Powerful evolutionary forces operating over millions of years have created, shaped, and maintained it. So it should not be too hard to imagine that this "social body" we live within is something of great importance to each of us.

Biological evolution mandates many separate factors in our survival—adequate amounts of oxygen, water, and forty different types of nutrients. Similarly, biological survival also seems closely linked to social needs. So where we stand in our society, how we get along with our spouse, parents, children, coworkers, the attention we give them, and the attention they give us, all are translated, transformed, and transmuted directly and indirectly by brain mechanisms into changes in hormone levels, shifts in neurotransmitters, signals to move and to stop moving, to attack and to embrace, to sickness and to health, to life and to death.

The emergence of our need for social organization is embodied in our bones: We have an upright posture and a thicker pelvis because of it. It is in our customs, such as why we use tools and the way we relate in sex. There is a set of distinctive features of the human animal, features which set us off from other species. Not our featherlessness, not the nature of our skin, not light beer, but some more fundamental forms of the human adaptation. Most of these are ignored both in medicine and psychology, where the built-in wisdom of our inherited traits is grossly underestimated.

Most of our friends and many of our colleagues and coworkers walk on their two hind legs, while most other animals do not. Humans are bipedal, which means we walk on two feet instead of all four. Chimps and gorillas can stand upright at times, but when they move they usually do so on all fours. A fossil skeleton called Lucy, the first known hominid showing evidence of bipedal locomotion, dates from about 3.75 million years ago, about one million years before the use of tools.

Bipedal walking and running are extremely versatile kinds of movement. People can cover more varied and in some cases greater distances over time than any other animal. The great evolutionary biologist J. B. S. Haldane pointed out that we are the only animals that can climb a tree, swim a mile across a river, and can also walk twenty miles in a day.

As we will soon see, while our erect posture had some disadvantages, bipedal walking was probably our ancestors' primary adaptive advantage over other animals. It has led to profound changes in human sexuality, the bearing of offspring, and the creation and the use of tools, each one of which has dramatically shaped our social living and associations. From a "body mechanics" point of view the engineering changes in the limbs made other adaptations necessary, created some immediate problems because of the hasty "redesign," and allowed for still other developments.

With the freeing of the front limbs, the hind limbs bear the entire weight of the body. The human back was not originally "designed" to support upright posture (which partially explains why back pains are a common complaint). Varicose veins are a problem for us because the valves controlling blood flow to the legs did not evolve fast enough to keep up with the excess volume created by the upright posture. There probably wasn't the time or the need to do a proper job on us.

More central is the problem and complex of changes with childbirth. To support the additional weight, the human pelvis grew thicker than that of the great apes. The thickened pelvis made the birth canal, the opening through which infants are born, much smaller.

But here is the problem: While the birth canal was becoming smaller, the brain and head were growing larger. If there had been no correction for this new disadvantage, the human species would have eventually died out because of inefficient childbirth.

The "solution" was to have human babies born very early in their development. At birth a baboon's brain is about seventy percent of its adult weight, while a human baby's brain is twenty-five percent of its adult weight. Human children have the longest infancy in the animal kingdom; they are not as competent and independent as baby baboons or baby chimps. Within a day, baby baboons can hold onto their mothers by themselves. The human child is immature for a very long period, for several years instead of a few months. The baby is helpless and will die if not taken care of. So our social dependency begins at our very beginning and is a matter of life and death from the moment of birth.

Unlike that of other primates, the major portion of the human brain's development occurs *outside* the womb, exposed to and influenced by many different environments, events, and people. The social environment plays a much greater role in the development of the human brain than in that of any other animal. And because the set of experiences of the surrounding physical and social world is different for each person, the specific kinds of abilities each of us develops varies enormously. This allowed our ancestors to adapt to the different circumstances of climate and "worlds" they encountered, and also now allows the human population a specialization and an individuality unprecedented in other organisms. But it also leaves us unfinished animals without strong social connection to other people. We suffer when the link to others is broken.

Another important consequence of the early birth of human babies due to our upright posture is that a helpless infant requires at least one caretaking parent to survive. In other species, because a newborn can fend for itself within a relatively short time, the mother can almost immediately resume her place in the group, providing her young with food and protection for a short time only.

But taking care of a human infant is a full-time job. For most of human history, it has been the mother's job. In subsistence societies, like hunter-gatherers, a nursing mother would have had a hard time getting enough food for herself while caring for a child. But parents working together form an efficient team. The father can hunt for meat and bring it home to the mother, who stays close to home gathering fruits and vegetables.

Human fathers take a most active role in the feeding of their young and become attached to them. The network of social bondings forms early in human beings, in part due to the immaturity of the infant and the long period of helplessness. Relationships in the first few years have a special biological emphasis given to them, a special quality and a special importance for the survival of the child.

That special quality is called the "attachment" between the infant and the mother or other caregivers. Even a young infant can tell the difference between the mother and other people: The baby's eyes follow her more than anyone else, and it smiles more enthusiastically at her. By eight months, most infants have a strong attachment to their mothers. They smile, coo, and attempt to stay close to her. When frightened, they go to her and try to cling to her leg or demand to be picked up. As long as she is near, an infant feels free to explore.

At eight months, the infant often shows extreme distress when the mother leaves. When the mother returns, the child will often cling to her desperately. The child cannot be comforted by just anyone—only the mother or primary caregiver brings relief. This bonding and early attachment serves to keep the helpless infant close to the mother, where it can be protected. Infants who wandered too far probably did not survive to reproduce.

The attachment of the baby to the mother is an important event. It is probably an innate bond which develops due to the gratification of the infant's (but also the mother's social) needs, the infant's cognitive development, and the communication between mother (or caregiver) and child.

In his masterful work *Separation and Loss*, John Bowlby shows that strong attachments have a survival function. Because an infant relies for protection on his primary caregiver, it is safer for the infant to spend most of his time clinging to or close by the mother. Babies do not necessarily become attached solely to their primary caregivers, but to people who interact with them socially, whether or not they provide any caregiving functions. Social communication, language, handling, playing, all forms of "socializing" develop this attachment. The connection to others is stimulated early.

Bowlby also noted that separation from an affectional attachment such as the mother-child bond has three stages: 1) anxiety, disbelief, and searching for the lost one; 2) depression, withdrawal, and despair; and 3) acceptance and recovery.

These stages have physiological effects, similar in the first two stages to the physiological arousal of the flight-or-fight response. Matthew Reite and his colleagues implanted telemetry equipment in infant monkeys to record their physiology when they were separated from their mothers. On the first day, there was agitation and increased heart rate. A day later the infants settled into depression, marked by decreased heart rate and low body temperature. After four days, the physiological signs returned to normal. Similar attachments occur in adult human beings, although it is not under such strict genetic control. But the same agitation, the same arousal, and the same feelings of grief occur. And there are dire health consequences of losing a loved one—breaking attachments can affect the immune system, the heart, and more, though they return to normal later on.

The early bonding and social communication within a family unit is also favored by changes in human sexuality. Most mammals are sexually aroused only at specific times of the year. All female mammals, except human beings, are sexually excitable only when "in heat," that is, when ovulating and when they can be fertile. Female mammals other than humans have an *estrus cycle*—they ovulate only a few times a year; males are generally excited by a female in estrus, and a female can only physically receive the male when she is ovulating.

Since ovulation in human beings is "concealed," not signaled by changes in odor or behavior, it becomes advantageous to act uniquely in matters of sex: to have intercourse throughout the year and throughout each menstrual cycle in order to increase the chances of fertilization.

There are good biological reasons for the swelling pleasures derived from sex; they encourage sexual relations more often and thus increase the chance of conception, especially in a system in which there is no clearly defined estrus. You may have noticed that many human beings like to have sex much more than the demands of insemination and conception require. The pleasure each individual derives from the other in sex can lead to strong feelings of attachment or bonds. Again, there appear to be strong needs, deeply rooted in our evolutionary history, which reinforce the formation of social attachments.

The sexual bond, or pair bonding, is the basis of another human social innovation: the family. Human fathers often stay with, care for, and care about their families. (Even in these days of reduced child support, suits and countersuits, the human male's responsibility is generally far greater than other primates'.) The mother can care for several small children at home if the father brings home most of the food. While the social situation may have changed drastically in the past fifty years, the message to adapt to the new circumstances has hardly had a chance to work its way through any system, not the social, the biological, or the genetic. Again this seems rather obvious, but the family unit is basic and has been quite important to human survivability as a species.

For contrast, consider the reproductive plight of the female chimpanzee. She has a life span from eighteen to about thirty-five years (in rare cases), but because she bears almost all the responsibility for the care of her children—the nursing, the direct feeding, and the protection—it takes her about sixteen of her years to conceive and to raise just two offspring. This just replaces her and her mate and leaves no room for accidents, for starvation, for deaths from attack, for early deaths, and the like.

The result is that chimpanzees now have a crisis opposite to that of the human: They are unable to sustain their population.

Human beings have been very successful reproductively, of course too successful to suit current conditions. A human female could theoretically produce and raise a child a year from the onset of menstruation to menopause, and the *Guinness Book of World Records* currently lists a record of sixty-four offspring for one woman, while the most one could imagine for a chimpanzee would be five. The male record, presumably for both species, is far higher, certainly in the thousands.

Our problem now is to keep this enormously successful reproductive strategy, evolved in a different time, in check. For better or worse in terms of our survival in the modern world, this complex of sexual and social predispositions is quite important and quite deeply rooted in brain evolution.

Back to the human story: In a mating system governed by estrus, the female is available only during the mating season, usually in the spring, and then to as many males as possible. Mating in most other animal societies is preceded by sometimes violent and normally aggressive competition among males for the females in heat. Out here in California, we watch each year the ritual of the elephant seal, a magnificent one-thousand-pound species whose males fight almost to the death for the privilege of inseminating the flock.

With the replacement of an estrus cycle by a menstrual cycle and the emergence of pair bonding, this continual sexual competition among males is lessened in the human species (although it may not always seem so to people like Woody Allen!). Increased cooperation can take place, not only within the pair bond but also among members of a society. All human societies studied so far display cooperation, as defined at least by food sharing and a sophisticated division of labor.

Almost every human being begins life dependent on the mother or the "primary caregiver" in today's jargon and world. As individuals mature, they grasp increasingly complex networks of interdependence, from family to group to nation to the entire world. For example, hunting requires planning, division of labor, signals of a complex order, cooperative carrying home of the kill, and a sharing of the prize with those at home.

From the moment of birth, then, we seem to be prepared to attach to our parents for a far longer time than is any other animal, because we are helpless without them. But the human being in adulthood is just as dependent on others as he or she is in infancy, though dependent on a more elaborate level. For we do not exist without the stabilizing cooperative network of society, for food, for shelter, for the production of goods, and for information. Imagine trying to do it all yourself.

Later chapters present evidence about how excessive self-centeredness damages the heart, how our physiology responds immediately to having to communicate with others, and how a break in our attachments to others or to family can result in disease or in death.

We experience these feelings of separation from others strongly, as well—feelings which may have once contributed to the maintenance, even the existence, of society. We don't like to be apart from the group, so the experience of immediate pain and suffering or the grief of separation might motivate the hardier and healthier to return to the group to cut the unpleasant feelings. Observing the dire consequences in others might also strengthen the reproductive bond in those not suffering separation.

Being a part of a group also favors access to sexual partners; these individuals will be more likely to survive and perpetuate the species. Isolated individuals do little to favor survival and continuity of the group.

Given these powerful forces which have, deeply within us, shaped and shadowed our needs for social connectedness, we may be able to understand why the loss of someone close to us could get inside us, even into our blood cells.

CHAPTER TEN

MIND-MADE IMMUNITY:
On Grief, Lymphocytes, and Sharks of the Mind

*E*very day thousands of people receive the phone call they dreaded ever receiving: The voice of a friend, relative, or stranger informs them that a loved one has died. The circumstances may be violent and shocking, or the death may have been the expected result of a prolonged illness. In either case the stress can be shattering.

Initially there is the shock and emotional pain of the loss, followed by a cascade of life changes as the bereaved must learn to live without husband or wife, father or mother. The grieving may manifest itself in both psychological and physical symptoms as the person struggles to adjust to the disruption of a vital social link.

For decades bereavement has been associated with the subsequent worsening or development of health problems in the survivors. Increased rates of infection, cancer, arthritis, and scores of other disorders have hinted at an underlying disruption of the body's immune system, that complex network of cells and organs which defends the body. However, it wasn't until the late 1970s that solid evidence emerged linking severe psychological stress with measurable changes in immune function.

Since 1975, R. W. Barthrop and his colleagues in New South

Wales, Australia, have been systematically studying the effects of bereavement—not only the emotional consequences but also its effects on physical health and immune function. In their initial study they followed the lives of twenty-six surviving spouses of patients who were either fatally injured or who died from such causes as heart attacks, strokes, and cancer.

In addition to offering counseling services to the bereaved, they charted the transient changes in their immune functions in the weeks following the losses. Several measures of immune function were conducted on blood samples from the bereaved spouses and compared with control samples from the non-bereaved. They found that the immune systems of the grieving spouses were indeed weakened, showing lower activity of what are called "T-cells"—a type of white blood cell that attacks foreign invaders.

This study was the first to show, in human beings, a measurable depression of immune function following severe psychological stress in a real-life setting. The findings may also contribute to understanding the significant increase in illness and death following the loss of a spouse.

There have been more studies since this first one. A study at the Mount Sinai School of Medicine in New York City confirmed the Australian findings and went beyond them. Men who were married to women in advanced stages of breast cancer showed a similar drop in responsiveness of the lymphocytes immediately after their wife's death and continuing for the next two months. But the immune functions began to recover soon thereafter. Between four and fourteen months after the death, the husbands began to recover their immune functioning, along with the lessening of their experiences of bereavement.

But how does this happen? How can grief and bereavement "get into" the immune system? Is it something the bereaved do differently from others? Changes in nutrition, in exercise and in activity do affect the workings of the immune system, but the people studied whose immune systems were weakened did not change their exercise or nutrition.

One idea about the linkage in these cases is that the "stress" of the loss produces changes in neuroendocrine and autonomic system activity which in turn affect the lymphocytes. It is a common observation, one often thought irrelevant by many physicians, that in times of instability or confusion some people are much more likely to get sick. What has made this common observation difficult to understand is that the *variety* of illnesses after stress is so great.

The disorders vary in severity all the way from simple infections to cancer—almost everything in these people seems to fall apart. They have stomach problems, their cuts do not heal, they may be more likely to get the flu, may have more fevers and rashes, and so on; one trouble after another.

The immune system may be the central link in the control of many of these disorders. It may well be that the increased death rates for widows and widowers may be due to depressed immune functioning. This also suggests a common factor in "getting sick" with diseases, the weakening of the defenses within the immune system.

Other, more hopeful studies indicate that the way in which people cope with stress—whether they actively seek to challenge their situation, whether they become helpless—may influence immunity and subsequent disease. Immune function can also be enhanced by purely psychological methods such as suggestion, hypnosis, and conditioning.

Of course, the relationship between upsets in the social world and the impairment in immune functioning is hardly the whole story. In the past few years there has been an explosion of scientific efforts which are just beginning to study the many influences on the immune system, from laughter to empathy, from bereavement to anger.

For some time, these links between the immune system and the central nervous system were in the realm of "there is no evidence for that," the kind of academic argument that assumes because there are no data, this indicates there is no possibility of a finding. It is a kind of medical and supposedly scientific thinking that assumes that systems within the same body would not bother to talk to one another, and that the mind and the body, since they are studied in separate departments, are actually separated. However, the person is part of several worlds at once, including the social; the immune system and the brain join forces as part of the person's continuing struggle to remain stable, to adapt to new situations and to change as new challenges come to the fore.

So it should not be surprising as it was to many that the organs of immunity such as the thymus gland, spleen, and bone marrow are laced with nerve endings; that the cells of the immune system contain receptors for neurohormones, neurotransmitters, and neuropeptides all thought to live only in the central nervous system; that damage or stimulation of the brain can alter immune function.

At this point we don't need to get involved in the details of the anatomy, but there is enough evidence now to overturn the early viewpoint that nervous system functions are unrelated to immune system functions. The supposedly separated worlds of *psyche* and *soma* meet in these junctures, and if they are not one, at least they are in touch enough so they do not go astray.

The immune system has, in a real sense, its own mind and its own decision-making capacities. It is part of the same body that the brain minds, part of the integrated defense of the body, and is one of its organs; almost as another sensory system it receives governance, or at least instructions, from the brain, and it talks to the brain. It has its own memory as well, and it can, instantly, create new cells in countless combinations.

If the immune system were an automatic system, like the sense of balance, say, and did not adapt or learn, then it would be difficult to imagine how events in different areas of life could affect it. But the immune system can learn, as has been known for years.

There were many reasons why the evidence was ignored; some were the result of simplistic thinking and intellectual blindness—the immune system was thought to be an automaton of the body, running on its own, with no relationship to the brain, and certainly not at all related to experience. Some reasons were social and political; unfortunately the Russians were ahead of us in this research, which made it difficult for American scientists either to credit the work or even become familiar with it.

But it was there: in Pavlov's lab, where, in 1924, guinea pigs were conditioned to produce specific antibodies when they were handled by research scientists.

Fifty years later the Americans made the same discovery. Robert Ader of the University of Rochester, now one of the leading figures in psychoneuroimmunology, was working on another Pavlovian learning experiment—conditioned aversion. In this standard research paradigm rats were taught to avoid saccharin-flavored water by pairing the drinking of the water with a drug, in this case cyclophosphamide, a chemical which induces nausea and other unpleasantnesses.

The rats were first given the flavored water to drink and then injected with the drug that caused nausea. They learned quickly, usually after one trial, to associate the taste of the sweetened water with the nausea. Then the taste of the sweet water alone produced the nausea. But there was a complication which made the experiment difficult to continue. They also seemed to learn to die from drinking the flavored water, long after the drug was gone.

Ader wanted to remove this "complicating effect" from the study, so he investigated the effects of cyclophosphamide. In addition to inducing nausea, the drug also suppressed the immune system, making the rats more vulnerable. This was the point of the breakthrough: The rats had not only become conditioned to the nausea, but they also seemed to learn to repeat the effect of cyclophosphamide on the immune system. The rats had learned to suppress their immune systems in response to tasting the sweetened water. Ader repeated the work many times and found that the conditioned rats were more susceptible to a variety of diseases, indicating that the immune system was suppressed.

Other experiments demonstrated that it could also be enhanced through conditioning. Reginald Gorczynski used skin grafts from unrelated mice to produce an immune response to reject the grafts. At the same time he paired this rejection response with a sham skin graft. Later he was able to demonstrate that the mice mounted an enhanced immune response to the normally inert sham graft procedure.

Such experiments mean that the immune system can be trained to defend more vigilantly or to relax defense. That the immune system does behave and learn is probably one of the major discoveries in neuroscience of the 1970s, along with that of the endorphins.

Needless to say, Ader's publication of the report in *Science* was controversial, but the work has progressed enough now to have been the subject of a major review in *The Behavioral and Brain Sciences* with generally positive results. The research work of the 1970s has been extended in many directions, among them the finding that different varieties of immunity can be conditioned separately.

But we are getting ahead of ourselves. What *is* the immune system, where is it, and how can mental events affect it? The "immune system" is not a set of visible organs and structures as are the nervous system and the cardiovascular system. Rather, it comprises many different cells and molecules distributed throughout most of the body.

Although it does not look like it, the immune system has certain similarities to the nervous system; both are primarily concerned with responding to outside information and with the regulation of the body; both respond to a great variety of stimuli; both receive and transmit signals, which are either excitatory or inhibitory; both exhibit learning and memory. It has been called a "liquid nervous system," only a small exaggeration.

The immune system serves in some respects as an additional sensory organ of the health systems of the body. It must identify and recognize what is foreign—not of the body—and what is not. In this it works like one of our senses, recognizing specific molecules. The immune system is on constant alert, scanning the body for evidence of foreignness. When a foreign body is recognized, the whole system springs into action—a series of steps is triggered, like a cascade, which results in a chemical and cellular attack on the foreign invader.

"Antigens" are normally foreign cells or large molecules originating outside the body that stimulate the immune responses required to defend the organism. At the same time, the immune system must not attack the cellular and molecular constituents of the body itself. The ability of the immune system to recognize and keep track of millions of different substances is another of the everyday miracles of biology. However, the immune system isn't perfect: It can overreact to harmless antigens—as in allergies—and it can also fail to recognize the body's own cells, attacking itself—as in autoimmune diseases.

There are two major mechanisms of immunity: innate, or "natural," and "acquired." Natural immunity primarily involves general inflammatory processes for reacting to tissue damage. When most cells (distributed throughout the body tissues) are damaged, they release molecules that increase the permeability of the capillaries, thus allowing other cells and large molecules to enter the tissues. These include complement, a collection of enzymes which helps to neutralize bacteria and viruses, and interferon, a family of proteins produced by cells in response to virus infection to inhibit viruses from spreading by "replicating" themselves.

Acquired immunity is different. It works through a type of white blood cell known as a lymphocyte. Embryonic cells (later in life found in the bone marrow) give rise to lymphocytes which undergo further specialization: Some are carried by the circulation to the thymus, where they undergo maturation to T-cells (the t is from thymus). Other lymphocytes mature in the fetal liver and later in bone marrow and are thus called B-cells. The various kinds of lymphocytes are sharklike: They patrol the blood stream and are ideally suited for the recognition and destruction of a million different antigens.

Some T-cells are important for virus immunity; some are capable of suppressing both T- and B-cell activity; "helper" T-cells, constituting two-thirds of all T-cells, are crucial for antibody-mediated responses; and some T-cells are important in attracting and activating a variety of other cells involved in immune responses.

The other major cell types in the immune army include macrophages (Greek for "big eaters") which are large scavenger cells that ingest and destroy antigens, and natural killer (NK) cells, which attack tumors and virus-infected cells.

How does this system work? It is basically a miraculous process if you consider it, since the system has to patrol constantly and be able to make millions of duplicate cells upon demand. It can work this way because the sharklike lymphocyte mutates wildly very early in embryonic life and produces a vast range of cells, each one with different specific surface receptors. These cells remain available for defense against practically any kind of invader. Those that match antigens which are a natural part of the body are inactivated, leaving millions more to mature for later identification and elimination of foreign antigens.

The antigen by its own molecular shape automatically selects its worst enemy from an army of potential defenders. When the lymphocyte cell pool is exposed to a foreign antigen this happens in rapid succession: Those cells possessing the matching pattern reproduce and generate an instant and enormous clone of identical lymphocytes. These instant defenders are specialized for the production of specific antibodies, which combine with and inactivate the antigen. At the same time, other sensitized T-cells migrate to the source of the antigen (say, a tumor), where they secrete chemicals called lymphokines, which are toxic to the foreign tissue. Still other alarms are sounded, and certain secretions attract and activate macrophages and other white blood cells.

The state of the immune system is the center point of the resistance of the organism, and perhaps more important in the development of diseases than exposure to disease entities (viral or bacterial) or toxins. For example, some viruses, like herpes simplex, are always present in the body, but they only become active when something goes wrong with the immune system.

Cells that could become cancerous constantly circulate in the body, but in healthy persons they are routinely eliminated by the immune system. The "mutant" cancerous cells can only take root when some factor, either genetic or environmental, has suppressed the functioning of the immune system.

There is no single best measurement of the health of the immune system. Obviously, the absence of infections, cancer, allergies, and autoimmune disorders speaks well for the integration of the immune system. Scores of measurements have been developed to test different facets of the immune response. The number and types of cells in the immune system can be counted. The killing power of certain cells can also be measured. Skin tests for allergens (such as ragweed pollen) or delayed hypersensitivity reactions to infectious agents (such as the tubercule bacillus) can also be used to assess immune function.

However, one needs to be cautious in interpreting the significance of changes in such immune functions. For example, a decrease in levels of T-cells circulating in the bloodstream may mean a decrease in immune function, but it may also mean that the these cells have migrated from the bloodstream into tissues where they can become active. Similarly, reduction of suppressor T-cells may, in fact, result in augmentation of other components of the immune system. Finally, changes of immune function in a test tube may or may not reflect medically significant changes.

What happens if the immune system gets out of balance and either fails to work or works too much?

Consider the massive immune deficiency AIDS—acquired immune deficiency syndrome. AIDS victims show a variety of immunological abnormalities including decreased helper-suppressor T-cell ratios, lowered T-cell counts, possible hyperactivity of suppressor T-cells, and hyperglobulinanemia (excessive amounts of pathological antibodies). As a result of this extreme suppression of immune function, people with AIDS are unable to resist opportunistic infections and cancer. At present,

AIDS is almost invariably fatal. The available evidence suggests HTLV-III, an infectious virus, as a causal factor.

There is a less severe variety of AIDS, called AIDS-related complex (ARC), that only sometimes develops into AIDS. However, not everyone who is exposed to the HTLV-III virus develops ARC or AIDS. It seems conceivable that personality and psychological factors again play a role in who gets sick and who stays well, but we would expect these factors to be less significant in the case of such a strong attack on the body. AIDS is certainly one candidate for the proper use of the magic-bullet approach.

Sometimes the immune system does its job all too well, overreacting to otherwise innocuous substances and producing allergic reactions. For example, hay fever is the result of an overzealous immune system's reaction to the harmless pollen in ragweed. Allergic reactions can be extremely serious: A healthy young man is stung by a bee. Twenty minutes later, he collapses and dies. What happened? He was a victim of a catastrophic immunological misjudgment known as anaphylactic shock. This sometimes occurs when people are reexposed to an antigen to which they have been sensitized, triggering an explosive inflammatory reaction. In marshaling all of the body's resources to destroy the poison, the person is killed.

Men often complain of being allergic to their wives. However, usually they prove to be actually allergic to their wives' cosmetics. On the other hand there are documented cases of genuine allergy of wife to husband. In France, a young wife developed symptoms of anaphylactic shock shortly after intercourse. Medical tests indicated that the problem was probably not due to Freudian psychological factors, but to the fact that she was allergic to her husband's seminal fluid!

Normally the immune system attacks only "foreign" substances, having learned "tolerance" for substances and cells that are a normal part of the body. However, sometimes the self-recognition mechanism breaks down and the immune system malfunctions, producing autoimmune diseases such as rheumatoid arthritis, myasthenia gravis, pernicious anemia, acquired hemolytic anemia, and systemic lupus erythematosus (SLE).

An apparently healthy young woman suddenly develops a bewildering collection of symptoms: high fever, skin rash, joint pains, pleurisy, kidney damage, and extreme malaise. What's wrong? Laboratory tests reveal her blood contains antibodies to her *own DNA:* The diagnosis is systemic lupus erythematosus (SLE), and the prognosis is not favorable. The cause of SLE is as yet unsolved, and unless medical science discovers a cure, this young woman is as likely as not to die within ten years.

Here is what a specific case of lupus looks like: Jane appeared completely normal until age three. At that time, in association with the birth of a sister, she suddenly became a serious problem, showing aggressive behavior with raging temper tantrums alternating with periods of melancholy withdrawal. Her aggressiveness worsened with time, and four or five years later she developed a number of additional symptoms including persistent fever, swollen wrists and ankles, anemia, jaundice, and skin rashes. Shortly after admission to the hospital, she died of kidney failure.

SLE presents a bewildering range of symptoms that come and go so unpredictably that no two cases are alike. The term *lupus* is Latin for "wolf," referring to the characteristic ulcerations that eat away the victim's face. The skin lesions occur because something has gone wrong deep within the immune system. In lupus, the immune complexes run wild: They get into blood vessels and kidneys and interfere with blood flow, hormone levels, and cause the visible skin lesions. Organic psychosis and seizures frequently result from inadequate blood flow to the brain. Patients with SLE will frequently have periods of severe symptoms intermingled with periods of complete remission. Flare-ups of the disease may result from a variety of causes including injuries, pregnancy, excessive sun exposure, overwork, irregular living habits, and emotional upsets.

Both genes and personality affect autoimmune disorders. The debilitating joint pain and inflammation of rheumatoid arthritis somehow involves autoantibodies known as rheumatoid factor. The genetic factor is illustrated by the fact that family members of arthritics are more likely than the general population to have rheumatoid antibodies in their blood. To investigate the contribution of personality to autoimmune diseases, G. F. Solomon and R. H. Moos compared healthy female relatives of arthritic patients who either did or did not show evidence of rheumatoid factor. Members of the group having the rheumatoid factor were psychologically healthier than those without it, which perhaps explains why they stayed healthy in spite of being at risk for arthritis.

The immune system is a highly complex system involving many components. It was once thought to function (somehow) all on its own. It is now understood that the immune system is, if not directly related to mental states, at least intimately linked to brain processes.

But how do mental factors or even specific brain processes affect the immune system? The answer is hardly known as of now, yet there are many important and promising new indications. There are numerous connections between the nervous system and the immune system, making it possible to understand how the mind can influence resistance or susceptibility to disease. For example, extensive networks of nerve endings have been found in the thymus gland, an organ that plays an essential role in the maturation of certain cells in the immune system. Similarly, the spleen, bone marrow, and lymph nodes are richly supplied with nerves supporting a brain-immune system link.

The cells of the immune system appear equipped to respond to chemical signals from the central nervous system. Receptors have been found on the surfaces of lymphocytes for catecholamines, prostaglandins, growth hormone, thyroid hormone, sex hormones, serotonin, and endorphins. These neuroendocrines, neurotransmitters, and neuropeptides may stimulate the differentiation, migration, and activity of lymphocytes.

The structure and organization of the brain itself may influence immunity. Consider a more prosaic relationship for the moment: Astute clinicians have made the observation that left-handed people appear to have more developmental difficulties. This is not too surprising since learning and learning disabilities are clearly a function of brain organization and development. But left-handers also have higher rates of immune disorders and migraine headaches, an observation that is more difficult to reconcile with current views.

In order to explore the relationship further, Norman Geschwind and his colleagues at Beth Israel Hospital in Boston undertook several controlled studies of left-handedness. The specialization of the different halves of the cortex for different functions and for different thought is a well-recognized fact of the human brain. In most people the left hemisphere is specialized for language and the right hemisphere for certain spatial functions. The brains of some left-handers may be similarly organized, or reversed, or may even have what is known as mixed dominance.

In one study 253 left-handers were recruited by distributing questionnaires in a shop in London that supplies items for use by left-handers. A right-handed control group, matched for age and sex, was also selected. The frequency of immune disorders was 2.7 times greater in the left-handers, most striking for thyroid and bowel disorders. In another study, a higher percentage of patients with severe migraine were found to be left-handed.

The mechanism or mechanisms underlying these associations are not known. Geschwind speculated that the male hormone testosterone, which plays a role both in brain development and maturation as well as in the development of immunity, may be involved. He hypothesized that testosterone slows neuronal development in the left hemisphere, while simultaneously affecting immune development, and thus favoring later immune disorders. This remains to be investigated. However, the association of left-handedness and immune disorders provides further evidence of the intimate relationship between the brain and immune function.

French investigators have been able to demonstrate an involvement of the left cortical hemisphere of the brain in immune function. Gerard Renoux and his colleagues removed a portion of the left hemisphere in mice. This resulted in a decrease in the number of T-cells found in the spleen. No change was noted when a corresponding portion of the right hemisphere was removed. So there is evidence from more than one source that the two halves of the brain act differently on the immune system. We might speculate that the link, as mentioned earlier, is with the emotional (anger and negative) component in the left side of the cortex, but we should note that these studies were done with mice, in whom this relationship has not been found.

But the brain-immune system that has been most extensively documented is in the hypothalamus. It is perhaps the single most important center of the brain, since it controls eating, drinking, temperature regulation, and many emotions. It receives signals from all parts of the nervous system, and from most if not all the organs via the hormones in the bloodstream. It regulates shivering, temperature raising and lowering, blood sugar in the body;

it operates via remote control the lungs and the heart, and more. It is very strongly involved in emotional reactions. It also seems to regulate the immune system.

This relationship has been demonstrated in the classical manner: The surgical removal of certain areas in the hypothalamus leads to suppression of immune system response while stimulation leads to enhanced immune system response. In an early study in Hungary in the 1950s two researchers first sensitized guinea pigs to allergic substances. When the hypothalamus was lesioned, those animals did not respond to the allergen, while intact animals responded with standard violent allergic reactions. Later research revealed that damage to certain areas of the hypothalamus resulted in decreased function in the thymus gland. Recall that the thymus is responsible for the maturation of the T-cells, which control immune surveillance and antibody production.

More recent studies have revealed that not only does the hypothalamus communicate with the immune system, the immune system talks back. In 1977 Hugo Besedovsky recorded the rate of firing of neurons in the hypothalamus when an animal was challenged by foreign and virulent antigens. The rate increased greatly, indicating that information about the immune system is registered, if not organized, in the hypothalamus. The stronger the immune reaction, the stronger the brain response; also, since the hypothalamus controls the pituitary, the pharmacy of the brain, there were significant changes in levels of the neurotransmitter norepinephrine—all of which suggest that the immune system can change brain function and vice versa.

So emotional states which involve the hypothalamus and probably other parts of the limbic system may also "spill over" and affect the immune system. It may well be an accident that this happens, or it may have allowed the health system to evolve to respond to unstable bonds. We are not, as we have said, sure yet.

Given the links between the nervous system and the immune system, the observation that different kinds of instability in the social world can affect immunity becomes less farfetched. Upsets, physical and psychological, have been shown to result in the release of several powerful neurohormones including catecholamines, corticosteroids, and endorphins. These, in turn, have been shown to alter immune function. For example, corticosteroids are known to exert powerful immunosuppressive effects, so much so that steroids are widely used to suppress immunity in allergic conditions (like asthma and hay fever), autoimmunine disorders (like rheumatoid arthritis and SLE), and to suppress rejection of transplanted organs.

During certain types of stress the brain also releases endorphins. Psychologists John Liebeskind and Yehuda Shavit were able to stimulate the release of endorphins by delivering brief, mild electrical shocks to rats. They found a corresponding decrease in activity and tumor-fighting ability in natural killer (NK) cells.

But was this immune suppression mediated by the release of endorphins? An endorphin antagonist drug was injected into the rats. When the natural killer cells were then tested it was found their activity was restored, supporting the idea that the immune suppression was caused by endorphins. This explanation was also reinforced by the finding that natural-killer cell activity was also suppressed when the animals were given a dose of morphine.

But do such changes in immune function due to stress have any medical significance? Additional animal research does link stress and the development of disease, in this case cancer. Vernon Riley and his colleagues performed scores of experiments on a strain of mice which were genetically predisposed to develop breast cancer. In one series of experiments the mice were subjected to what was called, delightfully, "rotational stress," that is, they were spun on a record turntable at various speeds (from sixteen rpm to seventy-eight rpm). The researchers found the faster the rotation, the larger the growth in tumors.

Other studies suggest that animals exposed to uncontrollable stress had tumors which grew more rapidly than in animals exposed to stressors they could control. Rats were implanted with a tumor preparation and the next day experienced inescapable, escapable, or no electric shocks. Fifty-four percent of the rats receiving no shock rejected the tumor; sixty-three percent of the rats receiving escapable shock rejected tumors versus twenty-seven percent of the rats receiving inescapable shock. These findings are supported by changes in immune function.

Steven Maier and Mark Laudenslager studied the differential effects on immunity in exposing animals to controllable or uncontrollable electric shocks. One group of rats was taught that they could terminate a mild electric shock by turning a wheel in their cages. Another group of rats received a shock every time the first group did, but nothing they could do would control it. Immune function was assessed by the ability of the T-cells to multiply in response to stimulation and the tumor-destroying ability of natural killer cells. The results showed decreased immune function only in the rats receiving the uncontrollable shocks.

But are such finding relevant to humans? It seems so: There are scores of studies showing that various types of social instability and the lack of resources to regain stability are associated with subsequent illness. The variety of the illnesses and a few direct studies have begun to indicate a breakdown in immunity. For example, Stanislav Kasl and his colleagues performed a study in 1979 of the development of infectious mononucleosis in West Point cadets. All the entering cadets were periodically given blood tests to screen for the presence of antibodies to Epstein-Barr virus, the agent which causes infectious mono. In addition the investigators reviewed interview data about the cadets, which included information about their expectations and family backgrounds.

Each year about one-fifth of the susceptible cadets were infected, but only about one-quarter of those infected actually developed symptoms of mono. What predicted those who were likely to become ill? Cadets who had "overachiever" fathers and who strongly wanted success in a military career but were doing poorly academically, were most likely to develop symptoms. The combination of high expectation and poor performance was reflected in increased susceptibility to infectious disease.

More recent studies link the onset and course of virus infections with stress-altered immune function. For example, approximately one person in three suffers from recurrent infections of oral herpes simplex. In a recent study, eighteen persons (aged between twenty and forty-three years) with a history of three to four recurrent episodes of oral herpes per year completed a stress questionnaire at two points: once within three days of the first appearance of a lesion, marking the recurrence of herpes, and another time selected at random when they had no active lesions.

In the week prior to a recurrence of oral herpes infection, the group reported increased stressful life events, daily "hassles," and anxiety, indicating that the presence of stressful circumstances is associated with an increased likelihood of recurrent herpes lesions. Yet it is probably not the actual stress which brings on the herpes, some later studies have found, but the person's *emotional reaction* to his disease. If someone is continually depressed that he has herpes, this reaction itself keeps bringing it back! In a California study the T-cells declined when the herpes sufferers were feeling depressed and returned when the sufferers were feeling better about themselves.

Janice Kiecolt-Glaser and her colleagues at Ohio State University College of Medicine showed that even mild upsets—mild, that is, compared with the bereavement of losing a spouse—can have effects on the immune system. In this study, medical students were observed for their number of "life change events" (which we shall treat in detail in chapter 14) in the previous months as well as for loneliness. Both loneliness and the mild amount of life stress these students had (they were doing well on exams) were associated with decreased activity of NK (natural killer) immune cells.

Stephen Locke studied how anxiety and depression affect natural-killer cell activity (NKCA), a measure of cellular immune function, in a group of 114 Harvard undergraduates. "Good copers"—those who reported few psychiatric symptoms in the face of high levels of stress—had significantly higher NKCA than "poor copers"—those reporting high levels of both stress and psychiatric symptoms. Locke also found that poor coping in the face of stressful life changes may adversely affect immunity.

Stress appears to "gets into" the immune system in a variety of ways. For example, during a situation in which there are conflicting signals—a sudden, unexplained threat, or a threat that is beyond the organism's ability to handle easily—there is activation of the sympathetic nervous system. This results in an increase in the level of circulating hormones that can suppress immune function.

Most of the research on the relationship of psychological states and immunity has focused on stress-induced immune suppression. But can positive states of mind enhance the functioning of the immune system? This is the subject of a growing amount of research. There have been many extravagant claims made for the effects of "positive attitude" or "imagery" on subsequent diseases, but there is little hard evidence. Some of this results from the confusion of health-building with the removal of diseases. Attitudes which may predispose one to avoid a disease may have no effect after it has begun. So all the imagery in the world may not work when a tumor has upset the stability of an organism, but a positive attitude may well maintain the balance so that one does not get sick. There is evidence that an individual can voluntarily improve immune functions. Howard Hall and colleagues at Pennsylvania State University tried to measure the changes. Twenty healthy people from twenty to eighty-five, male and female, were given blood tests before hypnosis, one hour after and one week later in order to measure the response of the lymphocytes in the immune system to challenges.

They were then hypnotized again and told to visualize their white blood cells as strong powerful "sharks" swimming through the bloodstream attacking weak confused germs (this is not too far from the truth about lymphocytes). They were given a post-hypnotic suggestion that these "sharklike" cells would continue to protect their bodies against germs even when they were not thinking about them. These people did self-hypnosis two times each week and told themselves the shark story.

Not everyone showed changes in immune functions, especially the older people. But enough of the group did show improvement to make anyone think about the separate worlds of the "soft" mental images and the "harder" phenomenon of lymphocytes.

The younger people showed a small but real increase in the responsiveness of their immune system to challenge following the hypnosis and visualization. In addition, those people who were easily hypnotized showed increased *numbers* of lymphocytes after their hypnotic sessions!

These changes in immune functioning were small, but so was the experimental "treatment"—just one hypnotic session followed by self-hypnosis for a week. But if such a minor series of events can lead to real changes in immune functioning, what might be the possibilities of increasing our ability to control the immune system?

Janice Kiecolt-Glaser and colleagues have found that relaxation training can also enhance cellular immune function. Forty-five geriatric residents of an independent-living facility were taught progressive relaxation and guided imagery techniques three times a week for one month. Relaxation was presented to these residents as a way to become more active and to gain some control over their world. By the end of the training period the relaxation-trained group showed a significant increase in natural-killer cell activity compared to a control group and to a group which had only "social contact" visits from a college student. The relaxation group also showed significant decreases in antibodies to herpes simplex virus; this is thought to reflect improved control of the herpes virus by the cellular immune system. These relaxation-induced improvements in immune function were accompanied by better self-reported health.

Kathleen Dillon and her colleagues demonstrated a link between positive emotional states and enhanced immune function. Ten students viewed a humorous videotape (*Richard Pryor Live*) and a didactic control tape. Their levels of salivary immunoglobulin A were measured before and after each videotape. Salivary IgA is a type of antibody that appears to defend against viral infections of the upper respiratory tract. Viewing Richard Pryor's antics temporarily boosted the average concentrations of this antibody. Furthermore, the researchers found that those subjects who reported using humor as a way of coping with life stresses had consistently higher levels of salivary IgA prior to viewing either film. Therefore, while viewing a humorous film may enhance immunity, the effect may be short-lived. However, incorporating humor as a way of coping with everyday life may have more lasting beneficial effects.

A series of controversial studies by Harvard psychologist David McClelland and colleagues has suggested that the need to exercise power over others is related to differences in immune function and susceptibility to disease. In McClelland's view, the "need for power" is the desire for prestige or influence over others.

McClelland has reported that college students who were high in power-related life stresses reported more frequent and more severe illnesses than other individuals. They also showed elevated levels of epinephrine and depressed levels of salivary immunoglobulin A. As expected, lower levels of salivary IgA correlated with reports of more frequent illness. McClelland interpreted the findings as indicating that if a strong need for power is inhibited, there is chronic overactivity of the sympathetic nervous system which suppresses the immune system. Similar results were obtained in a more recent study of first-year dental students. J. B. Jemmott found that students reported greater incidence of upper respiratory infections following periods of high academic stress than after periods of low stress.

The immune system has recently been shown to respond directly to a break in the mother-infant attachment. Christopher Coe and his colleagues separated squirrel monkeys from their mothers at six months of age. Immune function (decreased antibody response and levels of complement and immunoglobulins) was found to be suppressed in those suffering maternal loss. However, this separation-induced immune suppression was less when the infant was placed in a familiar home environment or with familiar peers. Both environmental familiarity and social companionship were sufficiently stabilizing to the infant monkey to reduce the emotional and immunological trauma of separation.

There is another area of work on how feelings, expressed or not, are associated with immune functions and disease. One characteristic of lung cancer patients, noted by many clinicians, is that they suppress their emotions. Cancer patients also seem to ignore their negative feelings, such as hostility, depression, and guilt. In a recent study that compared long-term survivors of breast cancer with those who do not survive, L. Derogatis and colleagues found the same pattern. The long-term survivors express much higher levels of anxiety, hostility, alienation, and other negative emotions than short-term survivors. They have more negative moods and expressed more negative attitudes toward their illness.

Norman Cousins, who has written extensively on attitude and emotions in health, recently recounted his experience visiting a self-help health group in Los Angeles. He met a striking-looking woman who appeared to him the essence of grace and dignity, like an older Grace Kelly. The woman had gone to her physician years before and was told that she had only six months to live. What did she say to the doctor? our visitor inquired.

She had told the doctor, "Go fuck yourself."

She related this to Cousins six and a half years after she was given her death sentence.

There have been a lot of studies on the relationship between expressing anger and breast cancer. In an early study S. Greer and T. Morris found that women who were later diagnosed as having breast cancer differed from women with benign breast disease in how they expressed anger. Those women who had breast cancer exhibited a greater amount of anger suppression and then sometimes extreme anger expression during their interviews. They held in the anger as long as they could and then let it out all at once. However, they mostly suppressed their anger.

These mastectomy patients, who had had an entire breast removed, were followed over ten years. Some of the women accepted their disease stoically. Seventy-five percent of these women were dead in ten years. Others adopted a "hostile and fighting" attitude. Thirty percent of these women were dead in ten years. There are, of course, many problems with this kind of evidence: The fighting women may have taken better care of themselves, and the sample is too small to conclude much from it. But the immune system is the system charged with marshaling the body's defenses to stop the tumor growth.

People who habitually suppress anger also have significantly higher levels of salivary IgA than people who are able to express it. Now, we are going far along here, but there may be the beginnings of a link between the effects on the immune system of lesions in the brain's left hemisphere, which may act like the suppression of anger, and the subsequent spread of cancer. It is unlikely that this will hold up, but viewing the brain as a body organ does lead into a different approach.

High levels of salivary IgA seem to correlate positively with the spread of breast cancer, which means that anger suppression may be strongly related to the spread of cancer. Greer and others, in a long-term survey, showed that women who responded to breast cancer with acceptance and feelings of hopelessness, those women who were quite willing to believe that the disease was God's will or something like it, had poorer outcomes than those women who reacted with denial or fighting spirit, as did Norman Cousins's acquaintance. Greer went back and looked at these women three years later and found the same results.

In a prospective study on breast cancer, Derogatis found similar results. Again, long-term survivors had significantly higher scores for several negative feelings including hostility, alienation, guilt, and depression than did short-term survivors. The long-term survivors were considered to be "less well adjusted" and had many more negative attitudes towards their illness and their treatment and, as it has been reported, "interview ratings also indicated poorer attitudes towards the physician among long-term survivors"—meaning (reading between the lines of this technical paper) that they were angry with their doctors as well. The long-term survivors of cancer knew that they were stressed, and they communicated their distress, whereas the short-term survivors seemed to be less able to enter and acknowledge their problem.

It has been easy for many people to assume that, therefore, cancer is "all in the mind" and that anyone who gets it is somehow at fault. Perhaps the thing to do is just to have the proper set of images, and it will all go away. But this kind of thinking is one reason the real effect of mental factors on health is not yet too well accepted.

There is no sense installing a fire alarm once the house is burned down. Obviously not all cancer, and not all phases of cancer, are susceptible to mental forces. Barrie Cassileth and her colleagues found no relationship between attitudes and survival or recurrence of cancer for 359 patients (204 with advanced malignancies and 155 with melanomas or breast cancer). Of course, advanced forms of cancer may be impossible to affect by psychological or neural factors, as the strength of the disorder may have already overcome the resistance of the organism. Disease remediation is of a different order than disease avoidance.

That there is a link between "getting it off your chest" and reduced cancer is tentative, but fairly well established. Why this might be so is not. One link may be hormonal. Hormones can influence the growth of cancerous tumors, and since emotions involve sympathetic activation, ventilation of anger may alter hormonal levels in the body. These hormone changes may also influence the immune system, perhaps stimulating immunity. However, any firm link is yet to be discovered. While "venting" emotions may still cause difficulty in social situations, keeping feelings to yourself may be injurious to your health.

You may have noticed that we have been taking a somewhat controversial approach to interpreting many of the psychological effects on the immune system, looking not only at the attitudes, moods, and thoughts of individuals but also at their relationship to the larger social environment. The increased rates of death of bereaved spouses and people whose childhood attachments are broken cannot be fully understood as an individual reaction alone. It is probably not an adaptive reaction for the individual organism, but a manifestation of how the brain and body act as one unit, even though this may not always be best for the individual. Of course, the reaction *could* be adaptive for the population, in which the deprivation of life support could cause the person to die.

But there seem to be some mechanisms in animals and in human beings that respond to social needs—though we hasten to add that there are many other mechanisms that respond to individual and internal needs as well and that operate at the same time. When the sika deer suffer from overcrowding, many of the herd die more quickly even though they have adequate food. Maybe the same phenomenon is occurring within humans when the immune system cuts down resistance in the person who is no longer part of a viable unit, as in widowhood or in grief. It may be an accident of the close neural connection of the systems, or there may well have been some evolutionary selection pressures on this accident, but there are relationships between health and the social world that might well be considered from this simple perspective.

And a solid and stable connection to the larger social group, or to humanity, signaled by attention outward, may have the opposite result: improved resistance, as the person is probably more valuable as a connected group member. From our speculative viewpoint this may explain why almost all societies have developed social conventions emphasizing the same virtues, and why there is such an emphasis in most religions upon caring for others, being generous to others, and serving them. Perhaps one of the many reasons is that doing so is not only helpful to the entire community but is so to the health of the donor.

Consider, in ending this tour of the beginning links between psychological reactions to the outside world and immunity, another even more controversial study from Harvard. David McClelland reports that when college students were shown a film of Mother Teresa (a winner of the Nobel Prize for peace) tending to the sick and dying poor of Calcutta, their immune functioning (as measured by salivary immunoglobulin A concentrations) immediately increased and remained elevated one hour later. So if this study is repeated and the measures prove accurate, even *watching* a person engaged in a "selfless" act may affect the observer.

McClelland noted in an interview that the effect occurred even in people who reported consciously disliking Mother Teresa: "The results mean that she was contacting these disapproving people in a part of their brains that they were unaware of and that was still responding to the strength of her loving care."

We wouldn't necessarily describe it that way or build a castle on these foundations, but attention directed outside the dominant self-system seems to be important for many aspects of health. Even attending to a pet or a plant seems to have health benefits. We don't mean to be absurdly reductionistic and imply that all social norms are for health purposes, but one aim of social and religious communities over the millennia has been to keep their adherents alive and viable, to encourage health through specific diets and prohibitions, through cleansing rituals and other means.

Could attention to the larger group, away from our biologically primary but primitive focus upon ourselves, and away from the hostile reactions to others, be something we are also organized to reflect? All this is a lot of speculation on a little evidence, and it may well prove to be misguided in the light of future research, but scientists and physicians may well have to think differently about how closely we are related to others in order to understand us, our organs, and even our white blood cells. The immune system is hidden, and its reactions are long-term and subtle. But a similar pattern of the importance of social connectedness for health seems more evident in what happens to the heart, worn by some on their sleeves.

CHAPTER ELEVEN

PRESSURE:
Social and Blood

When a person loses the stable connection with others in society, he or she feels it strongly: It may be experienced as loneliness, embarrassment, or hostility to others. But something else happens when there is estrangement: The heart, too, can break when there are breaks in social connections. A broken heart can result from the loss of a loved one, the loss of contact with one's feelings, or from feelings of anger and envy toward another person who is getting ahead of us.

These experiences can cause the heart to degenerate in different ways: The increased pressure in the bloodstream over time can tear the fabric of the blood vessels, and chronic hostility and self-centeredness can in some cases cause centers within the frontal lobes to send out a death signal to the heart.

The links between loneliness, companionship, attachment, or disconnection from others and the changes in internal physiology are made in the brain. Blaise Pascal wrote in 1670, "*La coeur a ses raisons qui la raison ne connait pas*" ("The heart has reasons that reason knows not"). This has stood for centuries as the description of the relationship between the heart and the mind. It has now to be amended in the light of recent evidence. It is not the heart at all, but our multitalented brain which possesses different sets of reasons within its separated small minds; the conflict between these "reasons" can sometimes kill the person. As soon as the circulatory system was discovered, it was immediately suggested that the mind can have profound effects on the heart. In 1628, in *Exercitatio De Motu Cordis et Sanguinis in Animalibus,* Sir William Harvey, discoverer of the circulation of the blood, wrote that "every affection of the mind that is attended with either pain or pleasure, hope or fear, is the cause of an agitation whose influence extends to the heart."

William Osler wrote in his "Lectures on Angina Pectoris and Allied States" that he believed "the high pressure at which men live, and the habit of working the machine to its maximum capacity are responsible for [arterial degeneration] rather than excesses in eating and drinking."

These ideas have also been present in less celebrated circles. Fred Sanford, Redd Foxx's television junkman, whenever he heard bad news would clutch his chest and say to his son, "Lamont, it's the big one!"

And most people know that the heart changes rapidly and continuously, as different emotions are experienced. Consider this recent report in which Dr. Thomas Graboys describes a patient who was an avid Boston Celtics (basketball) fan. Graboys monitored the patient's heart rhythm while he watched the Celtics in a very exciting final playoff game against the Philadelphia 76ers.

As the game progressed the frequency of the patient's irregular heartbeats continued until in the final minutes he began to experience episodes of ventricular tachycardia, a rapid, sometimes dangerous heart arrythmia. The Celtics won by one point, and it took nearly two hours for the irregular beats to disappear.

Every basketball game may need its version of the surgeon general's report from Dr. J.

James Lynch, professor of psychology at the University of Maryland, is one of the most interesting and important researchers studying the relationship of society, the heart, and the brain. In his excellent book, *The Language of the Heart,* he describes his intimate experience of the connection of the heart to the social body.

I suspect I first began learning about the complexity, the subtlety, and, even in some ways, the brutality of stress-induced cardiovascular reactions at a tender age. Even as a young boy, I blushed almost as easily as the wind blows across the open sea. Not the everyday, home-grown garden variety of blushing, mind you; not the subtle shift in color that you often see in people, a slight reddening around the cheeks and eyes, a charming glow. Nothing so merciful was in the cards when Nature wired my body. Whether it was the Celtic genes of my parents, the light coloring of my skin, a certain shyness, a deep-rooted sense of shame, hyperactive blood vessels in my face, an unconscious need to gain attention, an attempt to assault other people with my fiery face—or God knows how many other theories there are to explain it—the simple fact remains that back then as a boy and adolescent, and even today as a middle-aged professor in a medical school, when embarrassed I light up with all the splendor of a harvest moon rising to defeat the blackness of a frosty autumn evening. No pumpkin in all its resplendent autumnal glory could even begin to match the glow of my face when it decides to give me away.

Early in life I was forced to give up trying to be Gary Cooper walking fearlessly down some dusty street at high noon, determined to see justice triumph at any cost, showing not a flicker of emotion. Nor could I pretend that I was John Wayne surrounded by threatening enemies, standing tight-lipped while fearlessly commanding mere mortals not to be afraid. John Wayne or Gary Cooper, hell! I couldn't even walk across the floor in the eighth grade and talk to a thirteen-year-old girl during an Eddie Fisher recording of "Oh, My Papa" without my face lighting up like red fireworks exploding and sparkling in the darkness of a hot Fourth of July evening.

My firefly face was a dead giveaway. It was a fink, a bodily appendage that simply refused to hide my inner secrets. If I was embarrassed—bingo, on came the red. If I was angry, my chameleon surface quickly revealed me to the enemy. No one ever had to ask me what mark I got on a test: an A was gray-white; and F, bright red; and C—well, that was the usual color. If I was frightened, then I had to head for the dark.

. . . I secretly longed for the day when atherosclerosis would deaden my vasculature, when nature would give me its own rheostat to help modulate the glow of my face. But fantasies about the glories of old age could not sustain me, nor would my adolescent reality go away. Gradually it wore me down. I had to surrender and learn how to be comfortable being uncomfortable.

Almost everyone has had the experience of blushing. When someone says or does something that embarrasses us, or if we are caught in a lie, we blush. The blood vessels in the skin dilate rapidly. We feel a wave of heat wash over the skin, and other people present can see it distinctly reddening. It is most easily noticeable in the ears, but in people who blush easily and frequently, it can be a deep red clearly visible over the face, neck, hands, and all other uncovered skin.

No one blushes alone, and the act of blushing immediately connects other people to one's own distress. "I cannot recall ever blushing in the dark by myself, no matter what devilish fantasy was coursing through my brain. As near as I can recall, my blushing occurred only when other people were present. How often I wished it was the other way around," Lynch writes.

We blush only in embarrassment, either in a social situation, or later, alone, remembering what other people did, said, or might say—they are present symbolically. But if the act of blushing suggests so demonstrably that the vascular system is sensitive to the social world, could not the stability of the connection to other people cause other, and perhaps more dangerous, changes of heart?

It does, and Lynch points out that part of the problem causing high blood pressure is that people "blush internally" in social situations. External blushing is noticed by other people immediately; it demands a recognition or a response and is understood as a reaction to what others might be thinking of us. Maybe, he thought, high blood pressure is in part social: blushing inside.

Lynch's own blushing forced him to think about blood pressure, and when he did he began to notice that there were surges in recorded blood pressure when people talked. He was struck by the contrast between these hidden reactions (the blood pressure rises) and the person's apparent calm. Perhaps, Lynch thought, both blushing and blood-pressure elevations when people speak are communications to the outside world and within ourselves. They may be communications between the separate "brains."

These observations began an important line of research on the relationship of social pressure to blood pressure. Redford Williams found that when a person is talking with another who is equal in status, his or her blood pressure goes up very little. However, when a person is being interviewed by someone with higher status, either a physician or someone interviewing the person for a job, blood pressure goes up dramatically.

Lynch's own interviews with his patients suggested that the interview situation *itself* affects the cardiovascular output. Such experiences were by no means peculiar to these patients: Blood pressure taken in a physician's office is almost always higher than that recorded at home. An Italian study demonstrated that within four minutes of a doctor walking into a patient's room, the patient's blood pressure jumps higher, on average 27 millimeters of mercury systolic and 15 mmHg diastolic.

Might the higher status of the physician make one's pressure rise? If a person speaks to someone whose status is perceived to be higher, does that person's blood pressure tend to rise correspondingly? Relevant to this is the observation, often made clinically, that hypertensive patients frequently mention status problems in their jobs, have a lot of conflict with people in positions of authority, and often discuss their low self-esteem; so do they respond to status in a way that affects cardiovascular health?

Lynch and his research group studied forty college students with normal blood pressure. They were asked to be quiet, then to talk to an experimenter, to be quiet once again, then to read a book aloud. For half the students, the experimenter dressed in jeans and portrayed himself as a graduate student. For the rest, he dressed in shirt and tie and the laboratory jacket of a resident in internal medicine. He also told this group of students that he was an internist conducting a research project in blood pressure.

Blood pressure of all forty students rose when they spoke. The rise and the resting level of pressure, however, was significantly higher when the students spoke to the internist than when they spoke to the fellow graduate student.

If "social status" affects blood pressure of healthy college students, then is place in society registered in the bloodstreams of most of us? Are some people in low-status groups classified mistakenly as hypertensive and administered a risky treatment regime simply because they raise their blood pressure at the doctor's office? Perhaps they are not hypertensive in the rest of their lives, when they do not come into such stressful social contact.

Lynch wonders whether the significantly higher death rates from hypertension among black Americans and the disadvantaged are due, in part, to their low status in society. Are they frequently thrust into situations where they are "talking up"— that is, forced to communicate in a world where virtually everyone else is of higher status?

And what happens when one talks to those people who are lower in status? Consider, again, the pet phenomenon: Among people who had suffered heart attacks, a far greater number survived who had a pet at home than those who did not.

Lynch also studied the effect of the presence of a dog on the blood pressure of children when they were reading a book aloud. This was an unusual study in the way it was run, because Lynch, sensitive to the status and blood pressure phenomenon, asked his three children to be the experimenters.

The Lynch kids, who shared authorship of the paper, then went out and found neighborhood children and asked them to participate in the study, done not in the horrible, sterile, clinical, nervous-making laboratory, but in the recreation room of the Lynch home. Each child's blood pressure was measured (not, we might add, by the children) while sitting quietly and while reading aloud, both when a friendly dog was in the room and not.

The children's blood pressure was significantly lower, both at rest and while reading, when the dog was in the room. Another study, by Aaron Katcher, shows that people treat their dogs differently from the formal way they talk to each other. They speak to their pets more slowly and gently, and, of course, they pet their animals while talking to them.

Blood pressure is lowest when people are not talking at all, or when they are talking with someone with whom they are intimate, like their spouse. On the other hand, blood pressure is highest when a person is addressing a group of people unfamiliar to him.

Part of this rise in pressure, you might note, is a purely physiological reaction to the physical act of speaking. It requires a person to hold air in the lungs, increase pressure in the chest and abdomen in order to force the air past the vocal cords, and close the glottis somewhat to restrict the rate at which the air can flow out. This increase in chest and abdominal pressure can increase blood pressure dramatically. But this purely physiological approach does not explain why blood pressure varies so much depending on who is being talked to.

Deaf people, when they are communicating in signs, show the same rise in blood pressure. So it is not just the physical act of speaking that elevates blood pressure.

Watching two people have a conversation while they are both

attached to blood pressure monitors provides a rare opportunity to see an "interior" part of what happens in a social interchange. The blood pressure of the person talking almost invariably shoots up. That of the listener almost invariably drops. Even people with normal blood pressures send theirs up to what would be considered dangerous levels if the pressures were to stay elevated. In a hypertensive person, the rise is even greater, often to dangerous levels even in people on medication.

But what is blood pressure anyway, and why does it respond to social pressure? Blood pressure is the force (the "pressure") with which blood pushes against the walls of the blood vessels. When the heart beats, it pumps about three or so ounces of blood into the aorta, the major artery leaving the heart. The aorta divides into smaller arteries which lead into a system of tiny vessels —arterioles—which open and shut. The peak pressure, when the heart is contracting, is the *systolic* pressure, the low point, when the heart relaxes, is the *diastolic*.

Arteries squeeze their liquid content into the arterioles the way water goes through a hose: When water is turned on, it enters the hose, but if a valve at the other end of the hose is closed, the pressure in the hose will rise, and no water will go through. As you open the closed end of the hose, water flows out, and the pressure will then fall. In the bloodstream, the tiny arterioles are like millions of valves: When they close (*constrict* in cardiovascular lingo), the pressure behind them (in the arteries) increases. Blood pressure is determined by the amount of blood pumped from the heart ("cardiac output") and by the resistance the blood encounters in its passage throughout the peripheral circulation.

Blood pressure normally changes from heartbeat to heartbeat. People in whom the pressure is consistently high are said to have the disease hypertension. Hypertension or sustained elevated blood pressure has long been recognized as a leading contributor to a variety of cardiovascular diseases, including stroke and heart attacks: Hypertensives are two to three times more likely to develop coronary artery disease than are those with normal blood pressure, and four times more likely to suffer from a stroke.

Sixty million Americans are hypertensive, and about half remain untreated, a potentially dangerous condition because high blood pressure injures the blood vessels, which can later damage the brain, heart, kidneys, and eyes. Hypertension usually is not noticeable until there is a stroke, eye failure, or a heart attack, so it is often referred to in medical propaganda as "America's number-one silent killer."

Heart diseases cause more than 50 percent of deaths in the United States: Forty million Americans suffer from diseases of the heart and blood vessels. The economic costs of cardiovascular disorders, including loss of productivity and health expenditures, exceed $80 billion annually in the United States alone.

High blood pressure forces the heart to work harder; the increased pressure in the arteries can cause enlargement of the heart muscle, especially of the left ventricle, which pumps blood into the body. In addition, the high pressure and turbulent flow of blood can damage the walls of arteries, contributing to the establishment of fatty deposits, which can block the blood flow.

Such changes place the person under ever-increasing risk of a heart attack. In the brain, the constant strain of high pressure within the blood vessels can cause them to tear or to explode suddenly, leading to a stroke. Brain hemorrhages and other forms of blood vessel blockages are four times more common in people with hypertension.

Except for the few cases of hypertension which are due to kidney abnormalities, the vast majority of hypertension is called "essential hypertension," which means we do not know the essential cause. But the search for causes has been essentially restricted to normal physician's categories of "somatic etiologies" like too much sodium, too little calcium, too much of this hormone, too little of that. Hypertension is seen pretty much as a matter of the hydraulics of the system; the person has been by and large ignored.

What are the people like who have such high blood pressure? Lynch describes one such patient, a physician named Michael, who had dangerous hypertensive crises five years before he came into therapy. He had the classic symptoms of advanced hypertension, such as blurring of vision. His internist prescribed conventional antihypertensive medicines, which lowered his blood pressure but which caused side effects that were worse than his hypertension: sexual impotency and an overall feeling of loss of energy.

Michael had recently remarried after a painful and emotionally distressing divorce. Shortly after this second marriage he decided to stop using the medicines and run the risks associated with hypertension, in part because of the drug-related impotence.

Like many other hypertensive patients seen in our clinic, he seemed to be doing all the "right things." He exercised regularly, did not smoke, watched his diet carefully, and in general seemed to be in excellent physical shape. Yet his blood pressure was elevated up to levels that had to be considered alarming.

. . . He clearly understood the serious medical risks associated with sustained high blood pressure. He knew all about the sharply increased risks of having a heart attack or a stroke that had been linked to hypertension. He had seen more than enough pathology and sudden death in his clinical practice to question the seriousness of his own high blood pressure. His understanding of the cardiovascular system, and his clinical sophistication, had only made his struggle with hypertension all the more frustrating—or, as he initially said to me, "embarrassing."

His initial blood pressure was high, 170/110, well into hypertensive ranges; heart rate ninety beats per minute. He was calm about his abnormal blood pressure, calm "as a television newsman reporting 'live' from the scene of catastrophe." Lynch noticed the calmness and said that he would hate to play poker with Michael.

"Spent all of my life perfecting this smile," he countered, smiling. "It's worth a million dollars, you know. Patients love it. After all, you can't have your friendly family doctor looking unhappy and sick, now can you?" Glancing at the computer screen, which was tracing out the rise in his pressure, he continued, "Strange how I spent all my life controlling things. Do you know how hard it is to look at that? Just when I finally got everything under control, that thing goes out of control."

"That thing!" The phrase struck me as symptomatic of his problems with hypertension, and I repeated it for emphasis.

"That thing is part of you!" I then pointed out that his language was typical of the way virtually everyone disconnects medical symptoms from their personal selves. "Why do you think 'that thing' has gone out of control?" I asked.

He paused to reflect on the question and, while continuing to smile, quipped, somewhat sarcastically, "Maybe it's my arterioles? Or kidneys? Or the extracellular fluid system? Who knows, maybe my whole body has turned against me!" His voice then became more intense, his speech more rapid, and he stopped smiling. He alluded briefly to his divorce from his wife five years earlier, and the trauma it had caused. His adolescent children had great difficulty coming to terms with his leaving their mother, and their distress had been especially painful for him. Within sixty seconds his blood pressure rocketed up to 210/125, and his heart rate began to pound over 110 beats per minute. Concerned about the rapid rise in his pressure, I asked him to be quiet and breathe deeply. Within one minute, his pressure fell back to 175/108, and his heart rate to 85 beats per minute.

"That's amazing!" . . . "It seems that every time I talk about the past, that thing shoots up."

Every time Michael discussed his divorce, his pressure rose, as high as 216/139. He then stopped talking and watched the computer tracings of blood pressure and heart rate: "Thought I had gotten the past out of my system—but it appears what I did was push it out of my head and into the cardiovascular system. How do you control your own body when it revolts on you?"

He began therapy and learned to keep his blood pressure down to more normal levels without having to depend on drugs. Lynch's treatment program connects the person to an on-line computer, so that he or she can see how blood pressure and heart rate change while they talk. Lynch comments:

Seeing it all graphically plotted by a computer while he chatted with us led him to realize how totally disconnected he had been from his own body. He was, in turn, led to realize how completely unaware he had been of the feelings that went along with such major bodily changes. Simple conversations, and everyday social interactions that he had previously thought irrelevant to his problems with hypertension, were now seen as central to his disease. During the treatment, Michael learned that he had been disconnected from far more than an awareness of his blood pressure and his own feelings; he had been disconnected from his fellow men and women.

Lynch had great sympathy for his patients, because he now felt that his own blushed and very red face and all his years of continual social embarrassment worn on his sleeve may well have helped him to avoid some serious heart disease. The blushing was a signal to others of his strong feelings, and it probably forced him to understand and recognize them at the moment he had them.

For some people, those who might need Lynch-type therapy, their separated brain systems do not talk enough to one another;

the different centers seem independent. Others like Jim Lynch, less fortunate on a moment-to-moment basis, show other people direct red and bright signs of what they are feeling.

If Lynch is correct, that the link between human communication and blood pressure is strong, changing communication could change blood pressure. Lynch and his colleagues have developed such a treatment, which tries to link the social world with the one inside, and so is called *Transactional Psychophysiology*.

This jargon phrase is unnecessarily difficult, but psychophysiology is the study of the physiology of different psychological experiences, brain wave changes, heart changes, sweating, and the like. "Transactional" means it is the study of how different people transact, that is, how they relate to and affect one another. It is a way of saying he is measuring how the heart responds to other people in society.

In the kind of therapy Michael had, a patient, say, a woman, comes into a room and is seated next to a table with a box-shaped automated blood pressure device and an Apple computer. The therapist attaches a standard blood pressure cuff to her arm. "Sit quietly for a few minutes," he says.

Then he pushes a key on the computer, and her blood pressure is shown to her on a graph on the computer's screen. "Now, talk about anything," he says to her. She begins to speak about the weather, and he again pushes a key on the computer, and her blood pressure is shown to her compared to when she was quiet, only two minutes before. It is much higher now, in the range for which a physician would treat her blood pressure aggressively with medication.

"Be quiet again," he asks. She sits quietly again for three minutes, and amazingly, when he pushes the key again, her pressure is back in the normal range. In successive sessions, once every week or two, for six months, she will watch her blood pressure response on the graph, compared to that of minutes, weeks, or months before.

She will learn how it goes up when she speaks rapidly and breathes shallowly, and how it goes down when she speaks slowly, pauses for breath and breathes deeply. She will learn subtle physical signals, too small to be considered symptoms, such as her forehead feeling tense, or perspiration on her upper lip, that warn her when her pressure is rising. Most difficult, she will learn to connect these subtle signals to her social interactions.

She will learn to change her interactions with people and situations which consistently make her blood pressure go up. In a sense she will learn how to have a healthy dialogue with herself and others, and how she is *a part of* a larger social body when she speaks.

CHAPTER TWELVE

A HEART APART:
On Self-Centeredness, Hostility, and Sudden Death

Acolleague wrote one of us a letter describing her meeting with a famous physician on the occasion of a symposium in his honor:

I was very excited to meet Dr. [Blank] and his family at the conference as I had admired his work and all that he has done for the improvement of surgical care for the poor for the past twenty years. . . . I was invited to the Blanks' home, and he showed me all his collections of paintings, rare manuscripts, rare books and curios from all over the world . . . soon my view began to change. After showing me the artworks he and Caroline [his wife] got into a discussion, it must have lasted for more than a fourth of an hour, and it was only about their insurance policy for their art and their security arrangements in the home and then it went on about their financial future. I was puzzled. Then his wife told him that she had forgotten to mail a letter that afternoon, while he was at the award ceremony, and Dr. Blank's sudden outburst shocked me: "Goddam it, can't I ever trust you to do anything. I tell you, I'm surrounded by stupid bitches!"

I didn't know what to say, but we went out to dinner and Dr. Blank was driving. He drove too rapidly and a policeman stopped us, and it was frightening [the writer is from Asia and is not accustomed to the sight of highway policemen carrying guns]. Dr. Blank received a "citation," and when the policeman asked for the documentation on the car, Dr. Blank could not find it quickly, and went through the papers again and again. I could see him almost explode before my eyes and I was frightened.

He yelled at his wife again, saying that she was so stupid that she couldn't put things away in any order. We went on to the restaurant and had dinner, but it was not pleasant for me.

And he wasn't around much longer, for the doctor died of a heart attack at age fifty-five. This man, who was doing so much for society through his profession, and also by his charity, may well have been lost due to the kind of reactions he had. People like him have been described, somewhat circularly, as having a "coronary-prone behavior pattern." Two San Francisco cardiologists, Ray Rosenman and Meyer Friedman, began a series of studies of this phenomenon in the 1950s.

They reported, in a now-classic work, that people with coronary artery disease are often characterized by time urgency, excessive devotion to work, excessive hostility, denial of fatigue, competitiveness, and a hard-driving nature. Rosenman and Friedman found that, after following 3,154 initially well men for 8½ years, that these "coronary-prone" men were twice as likely to get coronary artery disease as men who do not behave this way.

Type A's, as they described them, have been characterized as the overbusy type of person, the one who is always trying to do everything simultaneously. A later report from their group says:

> Type A's may be found attempting to view television, read a newspaper or trade journal, and eat lunch or dinner all at the same time. "When the commercials come on, I turn down the volume and read my newspaper," is a statement we hear repeatedly. It is not unusual for a Type A to view two football games on two different television sets as he irons a shirt or treads an exercise bicycle.
>
> One of our postcoronary patients is proud of having built a desk onto his exercycle, which is in turn positioned so as to allow him to view television. He thus is able to get his daily exercise, sign checks, read trade journals and also view television—quadriphasic activity. "My wife can always tell when some exciting football play is taking place. I pump the pedals so fast that she can hear it in the next room," he once proudly told us.

Type A behavior has been defined more formally as "an action-emotion complex that can be observed in any person who is aggressively involved in a chronic, incessant struggle to achieve more and more in less and less time, and if required to do so, against the opposing efforts of other things or persons." It is not thought to be a general "personality trait" like aggressiveness, but a specific kind of reaction to challenge—involving the person's aggressiveness, impatience, and time urgency, which they originally felt was central and important to getting a heart attack; they even called time urgency "Hurry Sickness."

Type B's (the other type, of course) are thought to be much more placid; they speak more slowly, they do not try to do several things at once, and, at least in the samples studied, are just as successful as Type A's. What are the two types like? There are certain professions for which being a Type A is almost a prerequisite. Driving a cab in a big city is one, in which cutting everyone off, racing to get more and more fares, is probably the best strategy.

The Type A Behavior Pattern is sensitively distinguished from its opposite, Type B, by the Structured Interview devised by Ray Rosenman and Meyer Friedman. Although many distinguished researchers, including Flanders Dunbar and the Menningers, had previously attempted to discriminate coronary-prone personalities, they were psychiatrists and had focused on traditional, content-oriented interviews and tests of personality. Rosenman and Friedman reasoned that, since Type A's are people who respond to challenge with hostility and time urgency, the best test would be to actually put them into a challenging situation and observe how much hostility and time urgency they displayed.

They designed the whole interview to be irritating. They had people take time off from work, come to their hospital, kept them waiting without explanation, and then had an interviewer ask them questions about situations that made them hostile and pressed for time. The questions asked how they responded to waiting in bank lines and supermarket lines, how they liked driving behind someone who was going too slow and whom they couldn't pass, and so on. The interviewer, contrary to normal interviewing style, pressed them, was not very interested in their answers, and was not reassuring, supportive, or engaging. The interviewer interrupted, challenged, irritated, and threw in non sequiturs.

As important as the interview's questions, however, is the challenging manner in which interviewers ask them; a challenge such as an implied criticism evokes vigorous and explosive speech in coronary-prone individuals. The interview scored more on the way that the person answers the questions than on the answer itself. In the interview Type A's finish the interviewer's sentences when he is slow, and they cluck to themselves when the interviewer feigns dodderingness.

The interview is scored 75 percent on behavior and 25 percent on content. The principal behaviors observed, on audio or videotape, are voice stylistics and body language. No one is a perfect Type A or Type B. Everyone is a blend of both characteristics, and a trained rater weighs the balance in coming to a final score.

The voice of the extreme A in this situation is very strong, with a lot of word emphasis, explosive, bombastic, like a machine gun, rapid, staccato, vigorous, and loud. The A tries to control the interview, jumps in abruptly when the interviewer stops talking, raises his volume to talk over the interviewer, and can't be interrupted. The Type A has clipped, telegraphic, speech, sighs frequently, and fills in the time space available with placeholders such as "um-hm" or head nods. The Type A sits in a tense manner, smiles a tight-lipped horizontal smile, and has a nervous laugh. Perhaps the hallmark of the Type A is that he can easily be provoked to describe a hostile incident with such emotional intensity that he seems to be reliving it.

The Type B speaks in a monotone, rambles, seems subdued and lethargic, speaks slowly and softly, is easily interrupted, doesn't raise his voice, and sits in a relaxed manner. The Type B smiles with a round mouth and laughs a deep belly laugh.

The following are from interviews furnished us by Professor Charles Swencionis of the Albert Einstein College of Medicine, first with a Type A man and then a Type B man.

Q—Do you ever feel rushed or under pressure?
Mr. A—At all times.
Q—How would your wife describe you, as ambitious and hard-driving, or relaxed and easy-going?
Mr. A—Ambitious and hard-driving.
Q—When your children were young, say around six or eight, did you ever play competitive games with them, cards, checkers, Monopoly?

Mr. A—Yes.

Q—Did you ever let them win on purpose?

Mr. A—No, I would beat the hell out of them. [Embarrassed.]

Q—You mean you would beat a six-year-old child?

Mr. A—I would play with you and try to beat you. I'm always competitive. I'm sorry, it's just the way I am.

Q—Are you competitive off the job?

Mr. A—Yes, everywhere. [Sigh, horizontal smile, tight lips and jaw.]

Q—When you have an appointment to be somewhere at, say 2:00, are you on time?

Mr. A—Definitely. I would always be there 15 to 20 minutes ahead.

Q—What's so important about being on time?

Mr. A—I can't answer that. It's just important.

Q—Do you resent it if someone else is late?

Mr. A—Do I. I hate it. [Emotional.]

Q—Would you say anything to them?

Mr. A—Yes.

Q—What would you say?

Mr. A—All according to the way I felt at the time. I'd say, "What the hell's the matter with you? Can't you keep your appointments? Do you have to keep me waiting?" [Loudly.]

Q—You would let them know?

Mr. A—Yes, definitely. [Angry tone.]

Q—Do you remember a time when that happened?

Mr. A—Yes. Just before my heart attack. I had to wait for my sister-in-law. I had called her up about an hour and two hours before and I told her, I said, "—, be ready." I had to come [about an hour's drive] and I had to wait about 20 minutes or so, almost a half hour. When she finally got to the car, I was muttering a few things. I was trying not to be too abusive, because my father-in-law was there, he's an older man. But boy, I let her know. [Angry.]

Q—What did you say?

Mr. A—I said, "—, I had to come here, I had to wait for you, can't you make it on time? What's the matter with you?" [Angry.] I said a lot of things I shouldn't have really said.

An interview with Mr. B., a New York City cab driver, may show a few of the differences. If ever there were an occupation designed to bring out the Type A in anyone, this is it. Swencionis must have found the only Type B cab driver in existence. Mr. B talks slowly, without word emphasis, in a monotone. He rambles, and there are long pauses between the questions and his responses. He lets us see how important personality is in processing the environment, in allowing him to make a Type B world from a Type A occupation.

Q—Do you enjoy the competition for fares?
Mr. B—No, that's an ugly aspect of it. The people who are in it. . . . That's not. . . . That's not what the business is about. Actually, subsequently, you're not going to make your quota on the one fare that someone else gets. You're not always up against it. You'll get the next one. The keynote, the whole success of operating a cab is just not to have accidents, so that your car is always available and rolling. . . . If you put the time in, then it . . . a certain average per hour that's just what it's about.
Q—What about the competition in New York to always get to the next space?
Mr. B—Well, that gets to you, but only in a delayed way, after you've been driving for 8 or 10 hours, you feel kind of spent, shot. That's how it gets to you. I can get around traffic. You have to be very aggressive to be a New York City cab driver. Otherwise you couldn't make it as a cabdriver.
Q—Do you enjoy it?
Mr. B—Yes, I do. [Flatly, no emotion, no anger.] You get to feel as though you could go through a keyhole after a while.

These distinctions between responses to an interview and the first studies supported the early observation that a complex of behaviors called Type A, or some of them, was more likely to be observed in coronary patients than in other individuals. This research then became the foundation for a major prospective study, the Western Collaborative Group Study (WCGS).

The findings from WCGS established the Type A pattern as an independent risk factor for coronary heart disease. The National Heart Lung and Blood Institute critically reviewed the evidence and concluded that the Type A pattern is a risk factor in coronary heart disease "over and above that imposed by age, systolic blood pressure, serum cholesterol, and smoking and appears to be of the same order of magnitude as the relative risk associated with any of these factors."

Extreme Type A's display physiological changes indicative of stress: For the technically minded, they are: elevations in serum lipids and triglycerides, higher resting levels of the hormone ACTH, reduced secretions of 17-hydroxycorticosteroids in reaction to ACTH, faster blood clotting time, and elevations in urinary and serum catecholamines under challenging circumstances.

Descriptions of Type A behavior lump together many different aspects of personality and coping: from extreme competitiveness to impatience, from aggressiveness to explosive speech. The description of the Type A pattern itself took on something of a fixed, inflexible pattern of its own. It is useful to consider how the pattern was even named. Meyer Friedman, in a recent book with Diane Ulmer, writes:

> I have often been asked how Type A behavior received its name. In 1958 when we had been refused funding twice for a study of "emotional stress" and its possible relation to coronary heart disease, I went to Washington to see whether I could find out what was going wrong. I spoke to Dr. C. J. Van Slyke of what was then called the National Heart Inst., who explained that because we used the term emotional stress in the title of our grant applications, they were always sent off to psychiatrists for review. These specialists apparently doubted that two cardiologists and a biochemist were equipped to study emotional matters, and refused funding. Dr. Van Slyke, who had himself examined our applications, suggested a small word change. "I believe you fellows are describing a behavior pattern, something that you've actually witnessed," he said. "Why don't you just label it Type A behavior pattern? That should not upset the psychiatrists." We did so on our third grant application. It was favorably received and funded.

But the idea of an encompassing and complete behavior pattern has not held up over the years. Not all the behaviors associated with the original description are really related to heart disease. For instance, the desire to do several things at once may well be only a logical way to increase productivity. The key is *why* someone would want to behave that way. Is it possible to distinguish between the Type A characteristics that are associated with coronary heart disease and those that are simply benign correlates of Type A behavior?

We also need to know—and this is the critical issue—how the Type A person triggers the reactions which damage the heart. The answer is by no means obvious. Perhaps Type A persons, because of their behavioral and psychological characteristics, have a stronger physiological reaction to a normal discontinuity or stress than do their Type B counterparts.

Friedman and colleagues showed that when faced with a variety of psychosocial and performance challenges, Type A individuals are likely to show higher blood pressure and (to a lesser degree) greater heart rate elevations than are Type B individuals. Limited evidence also suggests that such reactions are accompanied by elevations in circulating catecholamines (adrenaline, for example), which have been linked in both animal and human research to damage in the muscular tissue of the heart.

When the situation is very easy or extremely demanding, Type A's and B's are likely to respond in the same way. What, then, are the particular challenges that elicit the higher physiological reactivity of Type A individuals? When the situation is frustrating, difficult, moderately competitive, or needs slow, careful responses, Type A's are likely to respond with higher reactivity than Type B's. Studies find that Type A individuals retain contact with stressful situations—and persevere longer than do Type B's in the face of fatigue, task distraction, and initial task failure. But in the absence of physiological measures we do not know if, for example, Type A people are more accustomed to such situations and so experience little or no additional physiological stress and strain.

Type A's more frequently engage in stressful activities of their own making and/or act to increase the stressfulness of the environment. Compared with Type B's, Type A's set themselves higher standards, behave more irritably and aggressively when they are frustrated, respond to challenges with exaggerated effort and intensity, and avoid working cooperatively on difficult tasks.

While the original discovery of Type A stimulated a lot of research and established an understanding of the relationship of the mind and the heart, it is in more specific responses to other people that many of the current discoveries about behavior and the heart are being made. They give a different picture: It is the person who sets himself apart from the social framework, an island into himself, and acts in a hostile way to others who is at risk, not necessarily the extremely busy person.

The Menninger brothers, Flanders Dunbar, and others have noticed that people who have coronary artery disease are more likely than others to be frequently hostile. While the specific findings of research into this area are not entirely consistent, they do suggest that certain of the Type A characteristics, such as the propensity for easily provoked hostility, are more important indicators of heart disease than an individual's reports on whether his or her behavior fits the Type A pattern.

And an analysis of a subset of interviews from the WCGS showed that speed of activity, achievements, and job involvement were not related to coronary heart disease, while the potential for hostility, which showed up as explosive and vigorous vocal mannerisms, competitiveness, impatience, and irritability, were characteristics of people who had heart disease. Karen Matthews, in an analysis of the WCGS data, found potential for hostility and irritability to be one of the best predictors of heart disease.

This too, has been known for centuries. Dr. John Hunter, an influential English physician (1729–93) who suffered from both hostility and angina pectoris, noted the relationship between his emotions and his heart when he said, "My life is in the hands of any rascal who chooses to annoy me." Dr. Hunter died after a heated argument at a board meeting at St. George's Hospital in London.

Hunter's case was the first to be described in both its pre- and postmortem phases. Hunter's biographer, according to Friedman and Ulmer, played down the doctor's easily aroused hostility, describing his "temper" as "very warm and impatient, readily provoked, and when irritated not easily soothed. . . . He hated deceit, and he was above every kind of artifice, he detested it in others and too openly vowed his sentiments. . . . In conversation, he spoke too freely, and sometimes harshly of his contemporaries."

Free-floating hostility is thought of as a permanent resident kind of anger that shows itself with ever greater frequency in response to increasingly trivial happenings. It may remain undetected and unrecognized for a long time. Here is how Friedman describes, in slight paraphrase, some of the indications:

> becomes irritated or angry at relatively minor mistakes of family, friends, acquaintances; critically examining a situation in order to find something that is wrong or might go wrong; if you find yourself scowling and unwilling or unable to laugh at things your friends laugh at; if you are overly proud of your ideals and enjoy telling others about them; if you frequently find yourself thinking or saying

that most people cannot be trusted, or that everyone has a selfish angle or motive; if you find yourself regarding even one person with contempt; if you have a regular tendency to shift the subject of a conversation to the errors of large corporations, of various departments and officers of the federal government, or of the younger generation; if you frequently use obscenities in your speech; if you find it difficult to compliment or congratulate other people with honest enthusiasm.

The Type A is very good at hiding hostility by always finding excuses and rationalizations for his more or less permanent state of irritation; when he becomes angry at another driver, the other driver has usually been in truth, wrong. Some of these Type A's even successfully make a career of their worry and anger, crusading against the very real problems of society, in unions, in charities, in public activism. But it is neither their very many activities nor their time urgency that is the problem for the heart.

Friends of the hostile person may find that he is outwardly expressing concern about the poor or other social issues, while being inwardly preoccupied with his possessions, his insurance, his pension, his status in society, his income, his investments, and more, and becoming angrier than appropriate about everything. Anything can cause this irritable eruption. Horn-honking in traffic is a favorite pastime for hostile Type A's. But they do not like it much when it is done to them.

Dr. W. Gifford-Jones was driving with a hostile Type A surgeon who was slow to step on the gas pedal of his car after the signal at the intersection had turned green. "The result was a sudden and loud horn honk from the car behind us. Immediately the Irish temper flared. My friend jumped up, walked to the car behind us, opened the door, grabbed the keys out of the ignition, and with a mighty toss threw them into a snowbank."

Or consider these comments from another Type A:

"I do not believe that I have excess hostility; this is due in part to the fact that my intellectual, physical, cultural, and hereditary attributes surpass those of 98 percent of the bastards I have to deal with. Furthermore those dome-head fitness freak, goody-goody types that make up the alleged 2 percent are no doubt faggots anyway, whom I could beat out in a second if I weren't so damn busy fighting every

minute to keep that 98 percent from trying to walk ov
answer your question however, if I could curb my inate [si
[sic], humility and empathy for my fellow man perhaps. . . .

Theodore Dembroski, James MacDougall, Redford Williams,
and others, in a study of cardiac catheterization, found that those
with the most blockage of their coronary arteries were the people
who showed the most potential for hostility and also kept their
anger in. People whose hostility was easily and frequently
aroused, but who then withheld expression of anger or irritation
against others, even when such expression would be appropriate
or deserved, were the most likely to have advanced coronary
artery disease.

This is not to say that we all should be calm and take everything
evenly, quietly, nicely, and sweetly. Anger has its function; it
mobilizes people out of uncomfortable and wasteful situations. It
is certainly necessary to express such feelings from time to time
for a person to get what he wants, to drive obnoxious or threatening people away, or to "clear the air."

However, if a person engages in hostility (which is characteristic anger expressed continually or experienced too often) or negative judgments, criticism and the like as a way of life, he is
putting *himself* at risk.

Hostility is currently the most popular candidate in the search
for the destructive Type A component; it has been linked with
blood pressure reactivity, severity of coronary artery disease, and
death from all causes including coronary heart disease. But what
are the reasons for hostility?

Hostility tears the social fabric; a move toward isolation of the
person so thinking. Excessive self-involvement may underlie hostility. If a person is very self-involved and thinks of himself or
herself as better than others in many ways, this person is vulnerable to anyone who confronts such claims or who looks better
than he. Hostility may be a strategy for coping with such challenges by saying, "Who do you think you are to challenge me
like this!" To the self-involved, many events are the cause for a
threat: the success of a friend, the turn of the stock market, the
prospects for one's company, the insurance crisis, the pension
crisis, the art crisis, the crisis crisis.

A very few research studies have tried to link Type A and self-
involvement. Dembrowski and colleagues found those who were

hostile during the Type A interview used more self-references (use of "me, my, mine, I"). There are more such self-references in angry outbursts of psychotherapy patients than in usual speech. The "mine" expression is the aspect of the self that claims ownership—"That's my money!" When we begin to look at the world only through our own eyes, a viewpoint usually considered egocentric, it seems there may be consequences within the brain and the heart. In the Multiple Risk Factor Intervention Trial (MRFIT), heart-attack survivors had been less self-involved than those who did not survive heart atacks.

Howard Leventhal, Kent Berton, and Larry Scherwitz accidentally discovered that self-involvement affects heart disease. In their study, which was supposed to be about anger, students who were either Type A or B recalled an incident that made them angry and later described it. But the most important predictor of the heart activation was simple: It was the number of times the students simply referred to themselves. Self-involved individuals had the strongest emotional and physical reactions to challenge, they expressed anger more intensely, and had much higher blood pressure, again at levels that would qualify for hypertension.

Scherwitz and colleagues did a similar study of self-involvement in 156 male patients who were hospitalized to undergo a coronary angiogram. Angiography offers a picture of the blockage in each coronary artery—a good measure of coronary heart disease. Those who were more self-involved had more severe coronary artery disease even after the researchers controlled other risk factors (Type A, cigarette smoking, and blood pressure). The more self-involved patients were more likely to have had a heart attack and were also more depressed and anxious. The most self-centered people also had the most severe coronary artery disease, and if they had had one heart attack, were more likely to suffer a second.

Maybe people became more self-involved after developing heart disease? This was not the case. The relationship of self-involvement and the severity of coronary artery disease was strongest among those who did not have a heart attack nor had discomfort. And in an earlier study, Lynda Powell found that people with great self-involvement were more likely to have a second heart attack.

Blood pressure reactions to challenges are higher, too, in self-involved individuals. So the social view highlights two reactions that can damage the heart: separating oneself from others by acting in a hostile way or by becoming self-centered. But how does the self-centered or hostile individual get to tear his heart out? Self-involved and hostile people have higher blood pressure, and they may be "hot reactors"—strong physiological reactors to stress. Such a person responds to everything as a challenge, and it is studied by seeing how much blood pressure and other measures of cardiac activation increase while playing a computer game. *Breakout* may be dangerous to your health.

The intermittent outbursts of heart activity from the surges of hostility finally damage the heart. The surges of catecholamines and other brain hormones that occur during anger may contribute directly to both arterial injury and the deposition of plaque on arterial walls. Over time, repeated traumatic emotional reactions may also fray heart tissue fibers, which, in turn, may lead to disorganization of the cardiac circuitry.

Abrupt increases in the flow of adrenaline, caused by sudden anxiety or anger, are now known to constrict thousands of minute coronary vessels, requiring the heart to compensate by pumping in high-pressure bursts. The high pressure and the rapid release of the neurochemicals throughout the bloodstream, as we have seen, cause the damage to both the heart muscle and to the vessels themselves.

Scherwitz and colleagues speculate that it is not the activity of people that is dangerous to the heart, nor the hurry or the speed, but the selfishness that underlies it. They assert that "if individuals are ambitious, competitive, or time urgent for purely selfish reasons, they may be at greater risk than if they are ambitious or competitive to serve others or higher ideals." In our terms, the latter are those who are interested in maintaining a stable connection with the larger "organism" of humanity as a whole. This perspective would also explain why those people who can look outward at others, at a pet, at a plant, or at acts of selflessness, as in the study of the immune system changes of people looking at Mother Teresa, might be responding to a deeper need within our brains than we and they know about.

If the cardiovascular system is a mirror of the mind, people who are excessively self-centered are doing themselves harm. The "me decade" of the 1970s may have backfired. Self-centered, hostile people set themselves apart *from* the world rather than seeing themselves as a part *of* it. They are cut off from the normal give-and-take of social intercourse, and the result may well break their hearts.

There is a faster method of heartbreak, however, which by-passes the route of social instability reflected in long-term activation of the system, which may weaken the heart muscles and the walls of the arterial system. Extreme instability or upsets can do it all at once.

The hijacking of TWA flight 847 in the summer of 1985 claimed its first fatality within the first 24 hours. He was not murdered by the guns of the hijackers. He was not on the flight itself. Flight engineer Benjamin Zimmerman's father, hearing of the hijacking, died suddenly of heart stoppage.

Nowhere is the way the heart mirrors what is going on in the world of the person clearer or more tragic than in sudden death. Disruptions in social or personal stability, such as the sudden loss of a spouse or a friend, a shock, a disappointment, or an accident, cause the brain to wheel wildly between different reactions.

In 1971 George Engel of the University of Rochester compiled 170 newspaper accounts of sudden cardiac death. He saw an interesting pattern. In most instances the deaths were preceded by events that were impossible to ignore and that provoked a response of overwhelming excitement, despair, or both. Such anecdotes were long ignored, but as Engel comments: "The puzzling fact remains that, with only a little encouragement, many physicians in private conversations are quite ready to recount from their own private practices examples of patients who apparently died suddenly under [emotionally charged] circumstances."

Until recently, doctors did not know the mechanism by which people died suddenly due to cardiac arrest. There appear to be two major types of cardiac death. The classic heart attack (myocardial infarction) involves blockage of one of the coronary arteries by a blood clot or spasm of the artery. Usually the arteries are already narrowed by fatty deposits in the artery walls.

The other type of cardiac death occurs suddenly, often without evidence of severe blockage of the arteries or damage to the heart muscle. Seventy-five percent of those who suffer this sudden cardiac death have no previous history or evidence of heart disease. The specific mechanism of sudden death appears to be sudden ventricular fibrillation, a rapid irregular heart rhythm. The normal rhythm of the heart is suddenly interrupted, and the quivering, twitching, fibrillating heart muscle is unable to pump blood effectively. But the ultimate cause of sudden death may lie within the frontal lobe of the brain, when its response to confusion in the world makes its different *"raisons"* active at the same moment.

But let's first take a closer look at the nature of the different reactions regulated by the brain. How did they evolve, and what determines whether they are lifesaving or life-terminating?

Our ancestors, for whose use the systems evolved, lived in small groups in an environment that was stable for millennia or more. Any sharp changes in it were likely to be rare but very important upsets to the stability of life. A sudden thunderstorm after a period of quiet, a sharp noise in the distance, and the unexpected appearance of an animal outside its normal range signaled the instability of the world to the brain and that something had to be done and done quickly: a real emergency.

Although this is speculative, those of our ancestors who reacted immediately and strongly, perhaps like a strong cardiac reactor, to sudden threats might well have survived better than others. Someone who fled at every sign of an approaching animal would be more likely to survive than someone who was calm. The payoff of two kinds of mistakes is quite different: there would be less penalty for running from danger, for a false alarm, than for a lack of concern. In the first instance only time might be wasted; in the second, the organism might well be dead. So there is probably a premium on fast or even extreme reactions to threats, since the payoff for not reacting, while infrequent, might be injurious to health.

Recent research has begun to link the observations that Engel made of preceding emotional stress and sudden cardiac death. As might be expected, the brain is involved. In a set of studies which may revolutionize our approach to sudden death, James Skinner at Baylor College of Medicine first simulated heart disease in pigs and was then able to produce ventricular fibrillation merely by stimulating the brain.

His work involved probing the frontal lobe, in human beings the area where the brain assembles information about itself and which action to take. Here, too, the brain perceives stress and controls blood pressure. Skinner found that by numbing certain groups of frontal lobe neurons, he could render the pigs' hearts immune to fibrillation. The signal is not a simple one, but the product of an instability of the different nervous systems.

In one experiment Skinner injected into the bloodstream of psychologically stressed pigs the beta-blocker propranolol, a cardiovascular agent whose success in reducing both hypertension and sudden death rates in heart attack survivors has always been linked to its action on nerve cells of the heart. These beta-blockers interfere with the action of the epinephrine and norepinephrine. Clamping the coronary artery moments later—after the drug had time to affect the heart but before it could enter the cerebrospinal fluid of the brain—always resulted in lethal ventricular fibrillation. But if the propranolol was administered directly to the pigs' cerebrospinal fluid, all attempts at inducing fibrillation failed. In other words, propranolol, a beta-blocker that is thought to work on the heart, acts like a brain drug.

"We don't think beta-blockers work on the heart to prevent sudden death," Skinner says. "They seem to work on the frontal lobe, where they alter the transmission of fundamental nerve messages to the heart." Skinner has also deactivated parts of the hypothalamus that control fear. He can thus prevent limbic system messages about emergencies from reaching the heart. Doing so stops the wild cardiac activation and also lowers blood pressure.

Cardiologists at Columbia University have found confirming evidence that antidepressants—brain drugs, if you will—are also sometimes effective in controlling heart rhythms. Other studies have found that the particular violent and often hysterical Type A voice mannerisms can be reduced by beta-blockers, but this change does not affect the amount of Type A content that is expressed in an interview. The clear implication of these studies is that the speech pattern and speedup found in the Type A pattern may also derive from brain processes.

The circulatory system normally can remain roughly stable or can return to stability even after extreme disruption. Blood pressure returns to adequate for vital needs as soon as one lies down, or when regular breathing or forced restoration of breathing can restore the heart rhythm. But when the brain is alternately sending out signals to start and to stop, to relax and to attack, the heart is twisted and pulled two ways at the same time.

Sudden death, or vasodepressor syncope, typically develops when there is a possible threat and instability. The reaction begins with arousal; the heart speeds up, and the sympathetic nervous system is activated. There may be a great deal of uncertainty about outcome and also whether flight or giving up is the more adaptive emergency response. But as uncertainty mounts, the opposite reaction may occur as well: Conservation-withdrawal, with parasympathetic activity, may be invoked. The frontal lobe "self" cannot decide, and we get two incompatible reactions at once. The heart simultaneously speeds up, while the muscle's tone itself is inappropriately depressed. This condition is typical of a heart that is going to stop working. The output of the heart is no longer able to sustain arterial blood pressure, especially when the person is erect.

Blood flow increases to the muscles for flight while the muscles are simultaneously inhibited for withdrawal. Under conditions of extreme or conflicting stimulation, the stability the two emergency systems normally maintain may break down, and *both* systems become active, simultaneously or in rapid alternation with each other. Watch an animal under overwhelming stress: A dog crouches, trembles, moves aimlessly, barks, whines, salivates, urinates, pants, and sleeps suddenly, but for a second. When people are confronted with a sudden surprise they respond immediately in the heart.

Maria Zefferelli was 14. She watched the race nervously. Would Renato qualify for the relay team? Would he lose badly? He had worked so hard for this chance, training every night, giving up almost every weekend and evening for two years, running almost to exhaustion.

It was close. The results were posted up on the board. Renato had qualified, but Maria could see that something was wrong, her brother just lay there on the ground at the finish line.

Maria ran down from her seat to pick him up and congratulate him. But when she reached the track, the doctor looked odd, gulped, shuffled around, stared down looking at Maria's feet and could hardly speak. When he did he said: "He's dead, of heart failure. It happens all the time to these kids who train too hard." Maria didn't know what to do; she cried, she sweated, she suddenly laughed, she remembered all the training Renato went through, she fell down, got up, slumped, got up again and then tried to run away.

Maria collapsed and died.

So the same thing may happen to people when there are unexplained and threatening situations: Is it an earthquake? Should we flee? Is he going to kill me? How do I respond to her advances? I can't figure out how my boss feels about me. Multiple interpretations and multiple responses are, unfortunately, the norm in our world and are the norm within the brain's separate systems. And we naturally seek simplicity and stability by the design of our nervous system. But often, especially in the modern world, we cannot handle the ambiguity.

Perceived instability may kill, slowly in the self-centered who respond to everything as a threat, and quickly when there are extremes. It is not just the slow progressive wear on the heart, leading, as a worn tire might, to a blowout, but the brain that is the locus of sudden death in an unstable social situation. There needs, of course, to be a heart that is weakened, but this only increases the probability of death; it does not cause it. The brain just responds to too much difficulty and goes to the extreme.

Lynch's patients live with high blood pressure for their disconnection; the hostile or self-involved may come down with a heart attack; and those who do not possess the stable structure for stable actions in new and even shocking situations may suddenly die, because the brain can't "make up its mind" to deal with them.

Social support and a consistent set of beliefs may work their wonders in promoting health by embedding one solidly within a fabric of stable actions and reactions to many different situations; this cushions any shock or stress and thereby prevents it from being too seriously disturbing. If the cardiovascular system is really a mirror of the mind and the emotions, one who has established long-term, stable social relations and a stable place in the world has a little extra cardiovascular stability as well.

CHAPTER THIRTEEN

FRIENDS CAN BE
GOOD MEDICINE

S ocial connectedness is so basic and vital to human
health that it affects blood pressure, the incidence
of heart disease, and the intimate workings of the
immune system. Because it is so important it makes sense to ask,
how are we doing as a society in fostering this vital factor vital to
the health of the public? Not well. We are a society on the move.
We move to the suburbs and then back to the cities. We move to
seek education or new jobs. We take jobs that require us to be
like nomads. Even those who remain in one place are surrounded
by a continual flux of new neighbors. Many become rootless with
no sense of community, no sense of home. Our families are
smaller, our marriages shorter. Lifelong friendships are increasingly rare.

Even the design of houses and communities can undermine
social relationships. In the name of creating healthier environments, entire communities are destroyed, people uprooted and
forced to relocate. One of the best-studied examples of this social
disruption occurred in the urban development project in the West
End, a community of some twenty thousand located near the
center of Boston. Largely populated by people of Italian ancestry,

the community was a maze of old houses, densely packed, some in quite poor condition. But the social life was very rich.

In 1953 the area was declared a slum, and redevelopment began. A study of the people who were uprooted and relocated revealed a tragic picture. Many suffered what could be called a grief reaction; feelings of painful loss, mourning, depression, frequent psychological and somatic complaints, a sense of hopelessness. One might well wonder which would cause more ill health: living in a crowded, older neighborhood or being forcibly relocated with the resultant disruption of social ties.

Consider your own relationships and community. When was the last time you just "dropped over" to a friend's house unannounced, without an appointment? How well does your community foster such casual and informal meetings which form the basis of a tight-knit supportive community?

Unfortunately, casual contacts, and even intimate ones, may not provide sufficient support for people in times of need and life crisis. For example, a study of cancer patients undergoing radiation therapy showed that less than half could identify a *single* person with whom they could talk about emotional problems. Other studies confirm that even the most intimate relatives and friends do not support the need of widows to mourn their loss beyond the first few days after the death.

Further, social support is not a cure-all. Maintaining one's health is not as simple as four hugs a day or to smile and say "have a nice day" to everyone. In fact, relationships can have their negative side. The more family members or close friends one has the more vulnerable one is to experience the loss of a loved one. Relationships can be financially and emotionally draining; just ask the spouse of an alcoholic or children caring for invalid parents.

The great majority of people need a lot of intimate contact with other people—so one finds that being involved in a relationship, even a bad one, appears better than no relationship at all. An Israeli study of ten thousand marriages found that those who reported a happy marriage had lower death rates than those who said they were unhappy with their relationship. Other studies show that being married, whether satisfying or not, offers more protection than no relationship at all.

How great an effect does marriage have on health? Is it just one of those effects which interest statisticians? Consider this: It is well known that cigarette smoking has a strong effect on death rates, so much so that there is a Surgeon General's warning to that effect on every pack. The Hammond Report was an influential compilation of evidence on smoking, and its conclusions led to the Surgeon General's famous statement. However, Harold Moscowitz, a professor of biophysics, reviewed the data in this report and found that the effect of divorce was about the same as smoking twenty-plus cigarettes per day! The data were:

Death Rates For

	NONSMOKERS	20 + CIGARETTES A DAY
Married	796	1,560
Divorced	1,420	2,675

From this perspective, divorce may also merit a warning from the Surgeon General.

So divorce has a profound affect on health, but any event like marriage cannot be the same for all people. One profound difference in marriages seems to be between its benefits for men and its benefits for women. As the experience of marriage seems very different for men and women in our current society, so are the effects on the health of both married men and women.

Two psychologists write of this:

In contemporary society, and perhaps historically as well, women, particularly married women, take responsibility for keeping up the family and friendship ties of their households with correspondence, with holiday and special occasional greetings, and with little gifts and thoughtful actions. Most adult men find this kind of attention to network maintenance tedious, if not downright distasteful. As a consequence they usually have invested less in maintaining the ties, the links in the support network. And in old age, it is the woman who reaps the rewards of her investment. So long as they are married, the man shares in the dividends. Spouseless men, however, have the fewest primary relations in their support networks, and as a corollary, the fewest family members giving them support of all kinds. Perhaps this helps to explain why older men suffer more upon the loss of spouses than do older women and why the man's emotional recovery from widowhood has been found to be slower than that of women.

Marriage appears to be clearly beneficial—for *men*. Compared with men who are divorced or widowed or who have never married, married men live much longer, have fewer mental and physical illnesses, and appear happier. Divorced and widowed men also tend to remarry very quickly. However, married *women* have higher rates of depression than married men, perhaps because they are often restricted and may feel that they are "only housewives." Some psychologists feel that marriage may be actually harmful to women. Married women have higher rates of mental illness than married men, while single women have lower rates of mental illness than single men.

But married men react more strongly to the loss of their wives than do women to the loss of their husbands. Death rates for widowers are more than three times higher than those of widows.

Part of the reason for the difference in death rates after the loss of a spouse lies in the different social relationships men and women form, at least in our culture. As many investigators have pointed out, in American society male friendships are not lifelong but are related to specific situations: school chums, sports or fishing buddies, work colleagues. Men do not usually find their main emotional source of support in these relations, they do not usually have a close confidant outside of their marriage, and their friends change more often than do women's.

By contrast, women's friendships have, at least historically, been quite different. They maintain close ties with friends of youth, with their families, and they are more likely to keep up long and permanent friendships even after an old friend has moved or remarried. In this American women might be considered closer to the norms of those of Japanese society than they are to those of American men. They have more close, long-lasting confidantes, whom they tend to keep even after marriage.

So, given the genetic basis for bonding, which begins with the attachment of mother and child, there is an immediate physiological reaction to the loss when a spouse dies. But since the woman is more likely to have another strong social bond than the man, she is less vulnerable to the loss and is less likely to suffer in health from the pain of bereavement, an event that is quite significant for health.

For men the increased risk of illness following divorce relates more to the loss of a confidante, increased loneliness, and the loss of embeddedness in larger social networks that the marriage provided. For women the increases in symptoms and mental health problems after divorce correlates most significantly to the increased financial strain coupled with intensified child-care responsibilities. This isn't to say that divorced women don't suffer as a consequence of loneliness. However, because women tend to have a broader social network and confide in a variety of friends and relatives, the detrimental health outcomes of divorce are not as directly tied to these interpersonal losses as they are for men for whom their spouse was more often their only confidante and close friend.

If changes in social connectedness can have such profound effects on health, as the bulk of the evidence suggests, then can interventions be designed to take advantage of the observation that friends can be good medicine?

Strengthening the social support of widows has been shown to improve their health significantly following bereavement. In a study by Beverly Raphael two hundred widows were assessed within the first few weeks following the death of their husbands. Sixty-four of the widows were judged to be at high risk for developing disease or symptoms due to the lack of support they felt from family and friends, their previously highly ambivalent relationship with their husbands, and their concurrent additional life crises. Half of these high-risk widows received counseling and social support while the other half did not.

At thirteen months following bereavement, only a third of the supported group reported bad outcomes in terms of increased mental and physical symptoms while more than half of the unsupported widows complained of health problems. In another controlled study of 162 widows by M. L. S. Vachon and colleagues, the women who received emotional support and practical assistance from another widow (the "widow-to-widow" program) reported quicker resolution of overall distress following bereavement.

Human companionship can also effect the course of labor and childbirth. A study was conducted to see if the presence of an untrained companion during labor would influence the course of labor and the quality of the mother's interaction with the baby following delivery. First-time mothers were randomly assigned to a control group who underwent labor alone (except for infrequent checks by the hospital staff) and an experimental group in which the mothers received constant support from an untrained lay woman. The support consisted of physical contact such as rubbing the mother's back or holding her hand, conversation, or just the presence of a friendly companion whom the mother had not met before. The rates of complications during labor were strikingly different for the supported and unsupported mothers. Seventy-five percent of the mothers without support were removed from the study due to complications during labor or birth such as fetal distress, stillbirth, cesarean sections, and induced labor. Only 12 percent of the mothers with companions developed such complications.

With uncomplicated labors, the length of labor was less than half as long (8.7 hours versus 19.3 hours) for the supported mothers compared with the unsupported. Following birth the interaction between mother and infant was observed. During the first hour after birth mothers with companions were more awake, talked to their infants more, stroked them more, and smiled at the babies more.

How does such human companionship get into the body to produce such profound effects on labor? While this question was not directly addressed in this study, other experiments suggest that anxiety associated with labor may increase catecholamine levels (epinephrine and norepinephrine) which decreases the contractility of the uterus and may lead to slowing of labor and fetal distress. Human companionship, particularly when a woman enters the strange and frightening environment of a hospital, may help allay anxiety and facilitate labor.

The friendly support may be from an untrained stranger, but similar or greater benefits might be expected when a family member or friend remains with the mother throughout the labor and delivery. Ironically, the technological preoccupations of modern medicine, with electronic fetal monitoring rapidly becoming the standard of care, have often undermined or interfered with human support, an apparently low-cost and effective intervention in labor.

Interventions to strengthen social support can also improve compliance with medical regimens and decrease subsequent mortality. In a landmark study, D. E. Morisky and colleagues followed four hundred hypertensive patients for five years after an initial educational intervention. The interventions consisted of a five-to-ten-minute individual counseling session, a counseling session with the patient and a family member, and a meeting with a group of patients and their families.

The involvement of family members to provide social support and encouragement to adhere to the medical regimen appeared to have paid off handsomely. At the end of the five-year period not only were the experimental patients more likely to keep their appointments, maintain their weight, and maintain a healthier blood pressure, but they were more likely to be alive. The group receiving support had a death rate 57 percent lower than the control.

There is other evidence on the effectiveness of psychological support during stressful medical experiences. A review of forty-nine studies of interventions designed to support and prepare patients for operations revealed that such interventions could reduce the amount of time the patient needed to stay in the hospital after surgery on average by 1¼ days. The interventions included informing the patients about the procedures and what they might experience and teaching skills to reduce pain, as well as providing psychosocial support.

These supportive interventions were aimed at getting an individual to help the person cope with a stressful event. Other attempts have been made to strengthen social support in entire communities with important, but harder to measure, results.

The Tenderloin district of San Francisco has long had a reputation as a high-crime, red-light area with extensive problems of drug dependency, alcoholism, malnutrition, and suicide. The most visible residents are former prison inmates, prostitutes, drug abusers, and former mental patients who were discharged ("mainstreamed") from state mental institutions. The hidden population, however, are the thousands of elderly residents who live in the numerous single-room occupancy hotels of the area. These residents, numbering some eight thousand, make up one of the largest "gray ghettos" in the country. The typical resident, an elderly white male, never married, has few relatives or friends, and little contact with other people either inside or outside the hotel.

In 1979 an important project began to alleviate the problems of extreme social isolation, poor health, and sense of powerlessness experienced by the Tenderloin residents. Students from local universities offered free blood pressure screenings in the hotel lobbies and began to meet the residents. They built up rapport and encouraged the residents to attend informal weekly group meetings. Ten to twelve residents and two student facilitators would meet and begin to discuss common concerns: fear of crime, loneliness, rent increases, alcoholism, nursing homes, medical problems, and their own sense of powerlessness. Gradually groups were organized in seven hotels, and participants began to identify common themes.

In one hotel the residents decided to become a more formal group, selected a name, and encouraged wider attendance by printing invitations, at their own expense, and planning a large introductory party. Small support efforts were organized. When a member of the group would go to the hospital, he or she would now receive a card signed by all the members of the group and a visit from at least one fellow resident. Before the group was formed such visits were virtually unheard of.

When an elderly group member was assaulted on the street and didn't know where to turn for help, her fellow members responded by forming the Safehouse Project. Going from door to door, they recruited dozens of neighborhood stores and businesses, which agreed to serve as places of help in time of police or medical emergency. Each safe house placed a large decal in its window depicting a bird in the safety of its birdhouse.

The forty-eight safe houses were credited with helping to bring down the neighborhood crime rate by 18 percent in the following year. But perhaps more important, they stood as a visible symbol to the residents of the positive changes they could make in the community through working together on shared problems.

There are scores of individual examples of improved health from these intentional support networks, some deriving from direct, tangible aid and some from the indirect effects of social interaction and companionship. A study is now in progress following several hundred residents to assess the effects of these community interventions on social support and health.

And we shouldn't think that it is only the old, the poor, and the disadvantaged who can benefit from the deliberate attempts to increase social support. Meredith Minkler, one of the directors of the project from the School of Public Health of the University of California at Berkeley, recently said:

> What we had not anticipated as outside facilitators is how this experience would affect our own lives, and how important this group

identification in the Tenderloin would become for most of us. Many of the students, for example, had left families, friends, jobs, and other traditional social supports behind to come to Berkeley and begin graduate studies, and the experience of meeting on a weekly basis with a group of very different, much older people, whom they nevertheless found themselves drawn very close to, turned out to be a personally very rewarding one.

In a more controlled experimental setting, but still in a real-life situation, Bengt Arnetz and his colleagues in Sweden were able to demonstrate physiological changes in response to increased social interaction. They chose as their subjects senior citizens on two floors of a residence home. The floors were identical in all respects including design, nursing staff, and residents. Although some sixty seniors lived on each floor, there was little social interaction. Social isolation and understimulation were endemic among these seniors and identified by staff and residents as major problems.

A social activation program was begun on one of the floors. Interest groups in botany, art, music, and song were developed among the residents, and special outings were arranged. The intervention resulted in a threefold increase in social interaction among the residents, staff, and outside people. A variety of physiological measurements were made before the intervention and at three and six months after. When compared with the control group the socially activated seniors showed some significant differences.

While the height of the isolated seniors decreased, that of the socially active seniors increased. Whether this reflected the increased physical activity, better posture, or changes in bone metabolism in the spine of the socially active seniors is not known. But blood tests revealed significant changes in certain metabolic hormones. The more socially interactive seniors had higher levels of estradiol, testosterone, dehydroepiandrosterone, and growth hormone. (These so-called anabolic hormones are ones that tend to build the body up and may offer a protection and counterbalance to the effects of stress.) These preliminary findings indicate that increased social interaction in real-life settings can prompt measurable psychoendocrine changes which are consistent with more favorable health outcomes.

Another field experiment in a nursing home was conducted by

Ellen Langer and Judith Rodin. These social psychologists wanted to test the hypothesis that patients who felt some personal responsibility and control over their lives would fare better physically and mentally than those who remained in a more dependency-producing environment so characteristic of most nursing homes.

Two groups of nursing home residents similar in socioeconomic status and general level of health were selected. One group, the "responsibility-enhanced group," was told that they were competent people capable of caring for and making decisions for themselves. They were then asked to choose a plant from a large box and told that they would be responsible for caring for it. Members of the control groups were given a plant and told that the staff would take care of the plant as they would take care of the patients.

Within a few weeks, the investigators found a noticeable difference between the two groups. The responsibility-enhanced group demonstrated a greater improvement in a variety of measures of physical and mental well-being and exhibited a visible increase in activity level and social interaction. Even more dramatic was the finding that eighteen months later, the responsibility-enhanced group showed a mortality rate of only one half that of the control group (15 percent versus 30 percent). No data were available on how well the plants in the two groups fared!

Changes in the work, school, home, or community environment can eliminate barriers to a sense of control and social support. A study involving this approach is under way among San Francisco bus drivers. Preliminary findings suggest that the city bus drivers may be driving up their blood pressures by working in a high-demand, low-control occupation. The investigators have found exceedingly high rates of hypertension among the bus drivers. The rates of high blood pressure for bus drivers was 1.5 to 2.0 times greater than that of the control groups, with one of the controls being newly qualified bus drivers who had just passed their preemployment physical examination. Among black drivers aged fifty to fifty-nine, the hypertension prevalence was an astounding 78.8 percent, twice that of the matched preemployment group.

What is it about bus driving that drives blood pressure up? S. Leonard Syme, one of the study's principal investigators, thinks that social isolation and job stress cause the blood pressures to rise. In spite of being surrounded by people all day, the bus drivers are actually quite socially isolated. Furthermore, according to Syme, "The driver leads his life according to a schedule that, in San Francisco, cannot be met. There's no way you can drive any segment of the bus route on time even on a Sunday morning in a race car." Nevertheless, when the drivers are late, which they usually are, they get demerits from their supervisors.

Drivers try to beat the clock by skipping food, rest, and bathroom stops during their twelve-hour workday, all the while having to contend with the complaints and demands of annoyed passengers and supervisors. As a result, Syme notes, "By the time they get home, they're not fit to do anything but go to bed and then get up and do it again."

Syme and his colleagues are working on recommendations that might help prevent hypertension among the bus drivers. Involving the drivers in making more realistic route schedules seems to be a promising approach. Also being considered is improving the quality of social support for the drivers by moving the rest stops from remote, isolated parts of the city to areas where they can talk with their peers. Supervisors and managers may be willing to consider such changes because they recognize the high costs of sick days associated with job stress and hypertension.

Investigation into how social interaction gets into the body to influence health represents a new frontier. While the traditional focus of medical interventions has been the sick individual, interest and evidence are now mounting which support investigations into health and disease as reflections of social connectedness. Interventions to strengthen social support are appealing because they have the potential to promote health and enhance general resistance to disease.

Something has to link the world of the internal organs with that of work. Something has to link the world of society with that of biology. That the brain is that link between the social environment and such phenomena as hypertension, susceptibility to influenza, and cancer would have been difficult to credit, let alone comprehend, given the narrow view of science in the past decades. Only recently have we developed a sufficient understanding of how the brain works, the dynamics of the cardiovascular system, and the role of the immune system in disease to provide a base upon which links between social relations, mood, and states of health and disease can be explored.

People need people. Not only for the practical benefits which derive from group life, but for our very health and survival. Somehow interaction with the larger social world of others draws our attention outside of ourselves, enlarges our focus, enhances our ability to cope, and seems to make the brain reactions more stable and the person less vulnerable to disease.

Mind-Made Health

CHAPTER FOURTEEN

FEELING BORED, FEELING BLITZED

*T*he brain is designed to respond to an enormous array of information: from words to pictures, from body temperature to sunlight, from the charge of an emotional exchange to the charge of ions in the air, from nutrients in our foods to odors in the air. The result is that all sorts of unlikely and unexpected stimuli can change our behavior and bodily function. The position of the sun can affect riots. The incoming weather can affect crimes. Some people become profoundly depressed as the sunlight wanes during winter in northern climes.

For many of these stimuli the brain has had millions of years to learn how to adapt. Species evolve to suit their original habitat, but for almost all species other than humans, the adaptation is set in fixed physical structures and fixed behavioral patterns. Birds fly but don't swim. Salmon exhibit a homing instinct, but they don't choose to live in condos.

For human beings adaptation is more flexible and wide-ranging. We have gone outside our original home in subtropical East Africa and now live all over the Earth. We can live for brief periods even outside the Earth itself. From the moment our ancestors stood upright on two legs, we began to walk into new

environments, explore unexpected places, and create unanticipated environments. As a result, we have had to learn to adapt
to unprecedented challenges.

Until recently these changes in the relatively stable environments to which we were adapted were gradual. No longer. The
world we are creating is constantly and rapidly changing. Travel
that was once unimaginable, like visiting the moon, is now possible. Phenomena like nuclear power and nuclear weapons, un-
imagined by our predecessors, now threaten our existence. Our
species' ability to create (which needs only a lone genius or a
small group) can leap way ahead of the ability of the remaining
billions of us to adapt.

In a way, parts of the brain are rooted in the "ground" of our
and other species' inheritance, while the rest of us reaches up,
now literally, for the stars. This process of reaching out beyond
ourselves can break us in the middle.

We face new challenges, often equipped with a brain and biology suited to a different and stabler world. The flight-or-fight
response, which evolved to mobilize the body to cope with physical threats, is now regularly elicited by symbolic ones. Financial
difficulties, an unsympathetic boss, traffic jams, and unemployment are unlikely to be successfully managed by an outpouring
of adrenaline, rapid heart rate, increased respiration, dry mouth,
moist palms, and tense muscles. Some of these biological reactions are obsolete, or at a minimum, inappropriately elicited. Yet
because they are provoked by symbolic events we have a choice,
a degree of flexibility. Events that happen in the world are not
directly reflected in the brain. The brain processes, interprets,
and constructs a model of the world. And that model, constructed of our beliefs, determines to a large degree how we respond.

Consider the current popular view of stress. People are seen as
passive, helpless victims. Stressors of all sorts, from loss of a
loved one to loss of our car keys, attack us, resulting in disease
much as germs cause infections. The answer: Avoid stress,
change, and challenge. Yet stress does not result simply from
exposure to events in the environment. The way we perceive and
appraise the event, the availability and use of resources to cope
with the challenge, have more to do with the outcome than the
raw event itself.

Stress, and its negative impact on health, derive from a mismatch between *perceived* environmental demands and *perceived* resources to adapt. The role of the brain in these vital perceptions helps determine whether some people break down in the face of demands while others seem to thrive when confronted with similar challenges. The balance of demands and resources is critical. Indeed, we *need* a lot of new information, changes and demands for us to grow and develop. As we will see, the absence of change results in boredom, which can be as stressful as information overload.

In a sense the brain operates as though there were a set point for optimal information flow and change. The brain tries to regulate the information flow within a range to maintain the stability of the organism. When the amount of information is too low, the brain will attempt to increase stimulation by seeking novelty and sensation. When the flow is too great and chaotic the brain also has mechanisms to reduce and organize the input and restore stability.

The brain's mechanisms for adaptation can be overwhelmed and blitzed by too much change and challenge. The study of stressful situations began with men in combat who suffer extreme psychological distress, which may severely impair their functioning and even lead to psychosis. This was called "shell shock" in World War I, "combat fatigue" in World War II, and "acute combat reaction" in Vietnam.

Under combat conditions, a soldier may have to make extreme demands on his body, going without sleep, food, or shelter. He may be called upon to commit extreme acts like killing. Finally, he may see his buddies become injured, disfigured, or die and may fear for his own life. Four decades later there remains a high incidence of psychiatric and neuropsychological difficulties in World War II veterans who had combat stress for prolonged periods.

There are other, more natural, forces which commonly cause stress: Disasters, such as fires and floods, earthquakes, and tornadoes, put people in grave physical danger and often result in widespread destruction. These are obviously stressful situations, yet those that seem less unstable cause less damage to the person: If the danger is anticipated, difficulties may be lessened.

But it is hardly surprising that such major alterations in the external world cause major upsets within: Our biology is designed to respond to instability. However, for several decades, researchers have noticed a consistent connection between the stability and predictability of a person's life and subsequent illness. This is a very important finding and deserves emphasis. Simply stated: People are more likely to become ill after experiencing major changes in their lives. However, as we trace the history and development of this finding we will see that the link between stress and illness is more complicated than that.

In the 1960s, Thomas Holmes, Richard Rahe, and colleagues devised two questionnaires, the Schedule of Recent Events (SRE) and the Social Readjustment Rating Scale (SRRS), which measure "major life changes" a person has experienced in the recent past. These life events include "positive events" such as marriage, vacations, and outstanding personal achievements; "negative events" such as marital separation, death of a close friend, and jail terms as well as "neutral events" such as changes in work hours, recreation, or number of family get-togethers.

It was difficult to rate these events as to how stressful they were, so Holmes and Rahe simply asked a group of people how much adjustment these different events in one's life would require. They set marriage at an arbitrary value of fifty "life change units" (LCUs). The relative ranks are given in the table.

Ratings of Stressful Life Events

Life Change Unit Values (with ranking)

LIFE EVENT	AMERICAN	EUROPEAN	JAPANESE
Death of spouse	100 (1)	66 (1)	108 (1)
Divorce	73 (2)	54 (3)	63 (3)
Marital separation	65 (3)	49 (5)	46 (7)
Jail term	63 (4)	57 (2)	72 (2)
Death of close family member	63 (5)	31 (18)	57 (4)
Personal injury or illness	53 (6)	39 (8)	54 (5)
Marriage	50 (7)	50 (4)	50 (6)
Being fired from job	47 (8)	37 (9)	37 (8)

	AMERICAN	EUROPEAN	JAPANESE
Marital			
reconciliation	45 (9)	40 (7)	27 (15)
Retirement	45 (10)	31 (17)	29 (11)
Change in health			
of family			
member	44 (11)	30 (20)	33 (9)
Pregnancy	40 (12)	43 (6)	27 (13)
Sexual difficulties	39 (13)	32 (15)	31 (10)
Addition of new			
family member	39 (14)	34 (13)	18 (23)
Major business			
readjustment	39 (15)	34 (11)	28 (12)

The amount of stress a person experiences within a year or so is considered to be mild if his or her "LCU score" is 150–199, moderate if it is 200–299, and high if it is over 300 LCU. Now this all may seem a little arbitrary and even silly. But the empirical studies which followed were hardly that: People who scored highly on the number of life changes had more traffic accidents than those who scored lower; and children whose parents moved, divorced, or got a large raise had all sorts of complications including higher suicide rates. And, as in the studies of bereavement, people who experienced numerous major life events were more likely to suffer from a staggering variety of medical conditions such as influenza, heart disease, diabetes, leukemia, rheumatoid arthritis, schizophrenia, psychosomatic symptoms, and depression, as well as difficulties in pregnancy.

After this, many pop psychology and medical writers began to blame the life changes themselves for the increases in stress. Slow down, don't move, watch that divorce comin' up from behind, keep stress low. Maybe all one has to do is never go outside or do anything (and it is true that extreme phobics have less disease). But life events do not come with inevitable disease consequences in tow, so proclamations like "job promotions cause cancer" or "divorce is schizophrenic" represent a kind of pseudosomatic disease mentality.

Although these early findings were surprising and established a new kind of link between social stability and health, many researchers began to question the assumptions of the scale and the way it was used. Some of the problem is the simplified nature of any early investigation. Obviously, not everyone finds marriage in the same relationship to other events as did the original sample. The loss of a spouse is very different for men and women. For Americans, the death of a close family member is fifth on the scale, but for a European sample it is eighteenth. So people are not passive victims of life events any more than they are helpless in the face of germs. We have an immune system to defend us from germs and brain mechanisms to defend against too much change.

The transaction between us and the life events is more complex than had at first been appreciated. Negative life events like a death in the family are more strongly related to illness, positive events are only weakly related, and not everyone who experiences major life changes gets sick. The nonoccurrence of a desired event may also be stressful, as when a person would like to marry someone but does not. These life events are not necessarily discrete ones that occur only once or all at once but often take place over time, with far-reaching consequences for many areas of a person's life.

An unhappy marriage or poor working conditions are not really "events" *per se*, but may still be very difficult to deal with. These life strains can be a result of the way in which a society is organized and from a person's position in it. A society that accepts some unemployment ("for the greater economic good") assures that some of its members will be under great stress and perhaps ill health.

For all our concern with disasters, unemployment, even divorce, these supposedly highly stressful "life events" are relatively uncommon compared to daily hassles. What about all those frustrating, irritating, and annoying common events like traffic jams, foul-ups at work, arguments, losing or misplacing things, concerns about weight or rising prices, and the myriad of other daily hassles? Even major life events are accompanied by such minor concerns. Getting a divorce may be destabilizing not only because of the emotional loss, disappointment, and conflict, but also because there is an increase in the number of hassles: fixing the car, cooking meals, arranging child care, and so on. Studies by Richard Lazarus and his colleagues have shown that at least in the short term these minor hassles are better predictors of both psychosomatic symptoms and physical symptoms than are major life events.

Stress alone does not predict illness; perhaps positive events, uplifts, can balance out negative ones. A person with a very active life may have a lot of hassles, but he or she may also be doing something that gives a great deal of pleasure—as in the case of an athlete preparing for the Olympics. Trying to balance school and workouts, having enough time for dates or outings, watching one's weight, and scrounging up money to pay coaches and go to competitions may involve a lot of hassles. But, for an athlete, the sheer joy of mastering new skills, winning matches, and maybe being the best in the world more than compensates for them.

Lazarus and his colleagues devised an Uplifts Scale to assess positive experiences. Not unexpectedly, people of different ages and occupations have different patterns of hassles and uplifts. A. D. Kanner and colleagues found that college students were "struggling with the academic and social problems typically associated with attending college (wasting time, concerns about meeting high standards, being lonely)." And while the middle-aged subjects found pleasure and satisfaction primarily in their family and in good health, the students preferred hedonic ("fun") activities such as laughing, entertainment, music, and the like. Even though preliminary research has not be able to link uplifts with improved health, this approach may still be promising.

There are different physiological systems at work within us. When you are stuck in traffic and you can't get to your plane on time, your heart pounds, your hands sweat, your stomach churns, and you feel more alert. These reactions may be more appropriate to prehistoric than modern times. As a medical student in the 1920s, Hans Selye, the main proponent of the stress concept, noticed something that eluded his professors. No matter what type of illness a patient had, one thing was common to all —they all *looked* sick. There appeared to be a common pattern of physiological reactions to extreme change. Selye called this response the General Adaptation Syndrome and identified three stages. First is the emergency or alarm reaction which prepares the organism for immediate flight or fight. Then comes the resistance stage in which many of the physiological changes associated with the alarm reaction are reversed, and the organism has *increased* resistance to the stressor. For example, in one study

Selye subjected rats to prolonged cold. After five weeks of cold, these animals—having developed resistance—could withstand even colder temperatures than rats that had been kept at room temperature. The third stage, exhaustion, occurs when the body's ability to adapt runs out. After several months of cold, the rats lost their resistance and became less tolerant of the cold than ordinary rats. At this point they were very prone to sickness and death.

We know a fair amount about the mechanisms of the general physiological reactions of stress but are just beginning to understand the more specific ones. The emergency reaction is mediated by the sympathetic nervous system. Its synapses directly stimulate the heart to beat faster and peripheral blood vessels to clamp down. The principal neurotransmitters at these synapses are epinephrine and norepinephrine. At the same time, the sympathetic nervous system stimulates the adrenal medulla to secrete a great deal of epinephrine and some norepinephrine, which are thus doubly assured of reaching the target organs.

If the emergency reaction is extreme or long enough to bring on the general adaptation syndrome, the hypothalamus stimulates the pituitary gland to release ACTH (adrenocorticotrophic hormone) into the blood. ACTH stimulates the adrenal cortex to release other hormones, the mineralocorticoids and glucocorticoids. If mainly mineralocorticoids are released, the body has made a decision to fight. These hormones stimulate the immune system to attack the stressor. If mainly glucocorticoids are produced, the body has made the decision to peacefully coexist with the stressor.

It is important to remember that not everyone who is stressed becomes ill. In the early studies of the effects of life events, about 30 percent of the people with a very high number of life change units did not develop illness. In part to account for findings such as these, Selye divided stress into types: distress (from Latin, *dis,* meaning "bad"), and eustress (from Greek, *eu,* meaning "good"). Both kinds have a similar broad physiological effect—as clearly as we can determine now—but in general, eustress is less harmful than distress.

Why? It is the same reason mentioned earlier regarding the different effects that emotions have on us: Positive feelings are a sign that things are okay; negative, that they need attention. So we are primed to respond to distress. Euphoria is short-lived;

distress lasts a long time. The eustress of falling in love does not last long, though the less intense pleasure of being in love may. The distress of taking on a job one may not be up to, or of living with a dying spouse, may continue for years. On the other hand, falling in love with someone who is married to your best friend may be a problem; leaving the job that is causing such difficulties may well be worse.

The concept of stress needs to be modified since the outcome depends so much on the nature of the stressor (type, frequency, duration, intensity), the individual's appraisal of the stressor as a threat or a challenge, the resources at the person's disposal to cope with it, and the individual's need for stimulation and excitement.

From this perspective the brain appears to have another set point. Much as we have a set point which determines body weight, this set point is for the amount of information, stimulation, and change that is optimal for the organism. As people differ in the amount they weigh despite similar diets and exercise, so too people will differ in the amount of stimulation they need. What is stressful noise to one person may be another's Beethoven; what is delightful peace and quiet to one may drive another up the wall. And as the set point for weight may change throughout life, so too will our needs for stimulation and information.

So it is not a simple matter of too much life change or overstimulation causing stress. Lack of stimulation can also be stressful: Solitary confinement is regarded by most as torture. In the Middle Ages, lords of castles paid a high stipend to display their own genuine hermit on their property, a hermit who was contracted to live alone near the house, but who would see no one. While there were many takers for these positions, most people left the employ, even at the risk of starvation, so basic is the need for the right amount of social stimulation.

The brain regulates the amount of information as it does with temperature and weight. The brain apparently has a need for a certain amount of stimulation and information to maintain its organization. When there is either too much or too little, instability results and disease may follow. It seems we don't want to go too far from the course the brain has set, in weight, in activity, or in the amount of stimulation received.

The bored brain may be as damaging as the blitzed one.

God, I hated that assembly line. I hated it. I used to fall asleep on the job standing up and still keep doing my work. There's nothing more boring and more repetitive in the world. On top of it, you don't feel human. The machine's running you, you're not running it.

As the brain evolved, its ability to handle the world became increasingly comprehensive. It developed increasingly sophisticated cortical and subcortical systems for receiving, decoding, analyzing, and reducing the varied and complicated flow of information. And the individual brain follows a similar pattern of development throughout the life span. Remember at age five or so what a triumph it was to know what a letter like *a* meant, then to discover that these letters go together to make whole words, and later that words go together to make sentences, sentences go together to make paragraphs, and paragraphs go together to make articles or books. But when one is older one can sit reading the newspaper for half an hour, and when the question comes "What's in the paper today?" answer, "Nothing, really." The world becomes organized, automatized, and familiar.

The paradox is that as the human brain matures and develops it both enormously increases its ability to find out new things and, at the same time, develops an enormous capacity for getting bored. It is easy for us to adapt to learn and to develop, and so we are in the crux of a two-horned dilemma—too much too soon, too little too late, both at the same time.

The brain of an experienced person in modern life is constantly attempting to achieve a stable balance of information and experience. On one hand we must deal with the destabilizing challenges of "life change," and on the other, the destabilization that can result when the brain is understimulated. Ours is a world that can become too familiar, too routine, with stop lights all the same, repetitive conversations, and stereotyped relationships.

Some attempts at change are adaptive. For instance, out of this need to stimulate themselves people have produced great works of art. Other attempts like thrill-seeking, fast cars, and drugs can be maladaptive. The cartoonist Sol Steinberg, discussing his art, said, "Avoiding boredom is one of our most important purposes."

Compared with one less experienced or developed, the more experienced brain does receive less sensory information because we have learned to extract out just those bits of information that we need. We need only catch a glimpse of a spouse's expression to know whether he or she is angry. We need to see only a tiny bit of a scarf on a chair to know whether someone is home. We need to hear only the beginning of someone's tone of voice to know whether we are welcome or not.

At each step we need less and less, we need attempt less and less. As we age we get more and more needful of strong stimuli. Young children are prone to be frightened by the unfamiliar stimulation, and they seem to enjoy repetition of the familiar more than older children or adults.

The maturing brain develops the capacity to better organize the world, reducing unnecessary information so that critical threats and instabilities can be recognized and responded to. This process of brain organization begins at the earliest moments of life. Even in the first days of life the twin tendencies of the brain, to seek stimulation and to reduce complexity, are apparent. Many psychologists have tried to characterize the perceptual world and predilections of the newborn. William James wrote that it is a "blooming, buzzing confusion." Jean Piaget characterized it as a transitory world: "There are no permanent objects, only perceptual pictures which appear, dissolve and sometimes reappear."

These characterizations are in part accurate. The world to the infant probably appears to be more disorganized than to the adult, and seems unstable and meaningless. Because the sensory systems are relatively well developed at birth the newborn's world probably consists of a sequence of sounds, lights, and other sensations, with less stability than adult perception.

In our view, the meaningful world of the infant may not be so much confused as it is simpler, more limited, than the adult world. Newborns are biologically unprepared to function and survive on their own in the adult world, but they are prepared to function in their limited one. Newborns are able to notice objects that are very close to them, things that are a part of their very small world. Later on, the newborns' world expands, and so does their awareness and capacity to organize it.

At birth newborns have the ability to focus at a distance of only about ten inches away, about the distance from the mother's breast to the mother's face. Later on, this range of vision and competence expands.

Newborns possess an innate set of preferences for moderate amounts of change and stimulation. In an important study, Robert

Fanz showed newborns a set of six discs. The babies looked longer at patterned discs than at single-color discs and longest at those with faces. At first they look primarily at the areas of most contour and change, the edges. At two weeks they preferred looking at a disc with a narrow, striped pattern to one with a solid pattern. Newborns need stimulation and surprises, but only in moderation.

It seems likely that the infant comes into the world with a predisposition to search out new features of the environment. And it seems likely that adults, too, have a "set point" for changes in level of stimulation, which may be different from person to person and from time to time in a person, but is probably an unrecognized dimension of experience.

The other side of our voracious organizational ability is that we become restless when things get too organized: We get bored, we need to change, we need to create something new. It was, in some part, curiosity and exploration that led our ancestors out of the trees and away from the savanna to every corner of the earth. We explore our environment as much to find stimulation as to find something in particular. Other organisms are also curious. Monkeys will work for the reward of the sight of another monkey. Indeed, even rats are motivated by curiosity: They will choose a more complex environment over a less complex one; they quickly learn to press a bar that makes a new compartment accessible to exploration.

Curiosity increases mental activity by conveying more stimulation from the outside environment. If you had to eat your favorite meal every day, you would soon wince at the sight of it. When one of us was in college, a friend of his had a job she was most excited about. It was in a candy store selling chocolates. She could eat all the chocolate she wanted, and for the first few days she was in paradise. After two weeks, however, she never wanted to see chocolate again! We are restless, "stimulus-hungry" creatures, even at the most basic physiological level of our nervous system.

Curiosity keeps us stimulated, but when arousal level is too low—just before sleep, in a boring situation—the level of performance suffers. Likewise, overarousal—being highly excited at bedtime, or restless when you are trying to study—hurts performance. Each of us has an optimum level of arousal. Many psychologists use an n-shaped curve (sometimes called an inverted

U) to describe this. The optimum level is in the middle of an organism's response range. Here pleasure is greatest, and reinforcement and the processing of information are most efficient. Some people cannot study without loud music on; they need to increase their activation level. Others cannot be in a room with any distractions; they need to decrease it. Working hard, exercising, resting, having a beer or cup of coffee, and turning music off or playing it loud are all attempts to increase or decrease arousal to the optimum level. The maintenance of the optimum level is achieved through feedback processes similar to the homeostatic mechanisms in the body.

People try to keep a stable level of stimulation going into their consciousness. It seems that different people like different "levels" of stimulation, as different people prefer their music at different volumes, or different amounts of spice in their food. Much research has been done on changing the level of sensory stimulation, since as you might expect, this changes consciousness. When a person is put into sensory deprivation, he will immediately try to seek stimulation. He may begin to move about, or brush his hand against his leg, or make noises vocally or with his feet. It seems that consciousness, accustomed to a supply of "news," needs its fix to keep going.

What happens when people are prevented from stimulating themselves? They rapidly become disorganized, lose intellectual ability and concentration, and their coordination declines.

Some, deprived of external sensory stimulation, begin to create their own worlds. Their hallucinations, according to one report on sensory deprivation experiments, are

> visual, often in vivid color and detail. . . . Virtually all studies are characterized by a range from vague or shapeless light sensations to complex objects and scenes, usually experienced in a progression from simple to complex. . . . Feelings of anxiety, irritability, boredom, restlessness, and unusual emotional lability are often reported, and paranoid-like reactions and alterations of body image are not uncommon.

However, the "disorienting" effects of sensory deprivation and isolation may be potentially beneficial. Sensory isolation has been used for relaxation and in smoking-control clinics. The radical shift in the environment may cause brain processes to change in line with expectations. There may be both pathology and benefit in boredom, depending on what we expect from it. For centuries meditative techniques have been used to reduce distraction from external stimulation; mystics remove themselves to a cave or to the desert, or they perform repetitive movements or sounds. The interpretation of these altered sensory experiences depends greatly upon the expectations of the subjects and of the experimenter.

Just as some people seek to reduce sensory stimulation, others go to great extremes to increase it. Thus people do strange, "sensation-seeking" things like riding roller coasters, driving quickly, eating very spicy food, jumping out of airplanes, going to horror movies, watching erotic films, and more. This shifts their arousal level to the high range of the curve, where even if it is unpleasant, the pleasure may occur later when that stimulation is reduced.

The brain constantly needs stimulation to develop, grow, and maintain its organization. It is not really a stable, fixed structure as the common view of the brain might suggest. In order to keep the organism going in a changing world, the brain has to constantly alter its organization, its circuitry, and even its neuronal structure in responses to the changes in experience outside. And it is responding to a much wider range of stimuli than we had thought.

The concentration of the neurotransmitters in the brain changes rapidly after a meal. A meal of eggs increases the available levels of acetylcholine in the brain. A meal that is rich in carbohydrates increases the brain's supply of serotonin. Neurotransmitters also respond to changes in the charge of small ions in the air. Hot, dry winds such as the foehn in central Europe and the Santa Ana of southern California are often associated with onset of symptoms ranging from irritability to headache and respiratory distress. Folklore concerning these "winds of ill repute" includes outbreaks of violence, even suicide, when these weather complexes prevail. Modern research shows that the occurrence of symptoms in weather-sensitive people coincides with a shift toward positively charged ions in the air.

On the other hand, air rich in negatively charged ions appears to have a refreshing and stimulating effect on us. Negative ions predominate around waterfalls, in clean mountain air, and at beaches, and disappear in polluted urban centers or enclosed spaces. The effects from minute concentrations of air ions seem to bypass the conscious part of the brain and work directly on brain chemistry and growth. Negative ions have been shown to increase brain serotonin, a neurotransmitter associated with more relaxed moods. In other studies, rats raised in a negatively ionized atmosphere had a cerebral cortex 9 percent larger than those in a nonionized atmosphere.

The brain is also light sensitive. Almost everyone experiences some change in mood related to the presence or absence of sunlight. On bright, sunny days we tend to feel better, perhaps more energetic and "sunny." On dull gray days, we may feel moody, blue, out of sorts. But for some light-sensitive people, the changes in light exposure may produce profound mood swings.

Consider the case of Mr. P., a sixty-three-year-old scientist who started experiencing unexplained depressive episodes at age thirty-five. After many years he began to notice a distinct annual pattern to his depressive episodes. Each year toward the end of June he would typically begin to become depressed. He would feel anxious, reluctant to go to work, and fearful of interacting with others. He had difficulty developing new ideas, and his sexual energy declined. He slept fitfully and became reluctant to get out of bed.

Mr. P. would remain depressed until about the end of January when he would switch dramatically into a hypomanic state. His energy level surged, and he required less sleep, sometimes as little as two to three hours per night. He had tried without success a variety of antidepressant medications.

Another patient, a twenty-nine-year-old woman, also suffered from depressions every winter and hypomanic episodes every spring. These episodes were curiously related to the relative latitude of her residence; the farther north she lived, the earlier in the year the depressive episodes began and the longer they lasted. On two occasions, she reported a complete disappearance of these winter blues within two days of arrival in sunny Jamaica. When she returned north after her vacations her symptoms resumed.

These patients are suffering from what has been termed seasonal affective disorder (SAD). This newly identified disorder is apparently not uncommon. The patients typically begin experiencing symptoms in their teens and twenties. The symptoms appear directly related to the amount of sunlight that reaches the brain. For people in the northern hemisphere the depressive symptoms usually start between September and October and last into March. One patient living in Chile experienced her depressive episodes between June and September, which are the winter months in the southern hemisphere.

Norman Rosenthal and his colleagues at the National Institutes of Health developed a novel approach to treating such patients. Reasoning that the symptoms were due to an extreme reaction of the brain to light deprivation, light therapy was prescribed. The patients were instructed to sit directly in front of a bright, full-spectrum fluorescent light source for three hours before dawn and three hours after dusk. A control group sat an equal amount of time in front of a dim yellow light. The antidepressive effects of the high-intensity light treatment were dramatic. The mechanism of action is not yet clear, but it is known that the brain, including its deepest structures like the pineal gland, is sensitive to the presence of light. Seasonal affective disorder provides a vivid example of the sensitivity, often unrecognized or dismissed, of the brain to various types of physical stimulation.

Visual stimulation can also effect our health. According to a recent controlled study of hospitalized patients, those who have a room with a view recover more quickly than those who stare out at a brick wall. Roger Ulrich from the University of Delaware studied forty-six patients who had undergone gall bladder surgery. Half the patients had hospital rooms with a window looking out onto a small stand of deciduous trees while the matched controls had a view of a brown brick wall.

The patients with a view of the trees spent fewer days in the hospital after surgery (by nearly one day), had fewer negative evaluations in the nursing notes, and took fewer doses of moderate and strong pain medications. They also had slightly fewer postoperative complications.

The view of a natural arbor scene appeared to have a decidedly therapeutic effect, at least when compared with a view of a brown brick wall. Whether similar salutary effects could be achieved by pictures or murals depicting outdoor scenes is not known but is worth considering. In discussing his findings, Ulrich remarks:

> The conclusions cannot be extended to all built views, nor to other patient groups, such as long-term patients, who may suffer from low arousal or boredom rather than from the anxiety problems typically associated with surgeries. Perhaps to a chronically understimulated

patient, a built view such as a lively city street might be more stimulating and hence more therapeutic than many natural views. These cautions notwithstanding, the results imply that hospital design and siting decisions should take into account the quality of patient window views.

Some unexpected bits of verbal information also seem to seep into the mind, indirectly, under the threshold of conscious awareness. The sleeping brain monitors the environment for meaningful sounds. We will awaken when our name is called but not someone else's. When sleeping people listen to recordings of names being read, they show a profound cortical response to their own names, and, again, not to others'.

A new series of studies by the psychiatrist Lloyd Silverman of New York University shows that subliminal stimulation does seem to have effects. In earlier studies it was found that when some words are flashed subliminally (too quickly to register consciously) to a person, those that are taboo (or were when the study was done) take longer to recognize. *Whore* takes longer, for instance, than *shore*. Also, people tend to develop specific feelings to stimuli even though they cannot recognize the source. When geometric shapes are flashed to the person faster than he can recognize them and the person is asked, "How much do you like them?" he likes those figures he has seen before, while insisting the question is nonsensical.

There are many other indications that we can react to information at a level below consciousness. Changes in skin resistance, heart rate, and other measures of activation may suggest that our brains and body may react to certain information we may not be consciously aware of. There is a growing, but still controversial, body of research literature showing that we may be profoundly affected by this "subliminal stimulation." The effects of these indirect stimuli are often indirect as well.

In an important series of studies by Silverman, the sentence "Mommy and I are 1" was flashed to a person who was unaware of the message. When groups who had seen this message were later tested on a variety of tasks, such as later achievement, exam scores, and aspirations, all performances seem enhanced. These studies were done with the idea of supporting the psychoanalytic point of view that the experience of such "oneness" will enhance performance. While it is not necessary to accept such a seemingly implausible idea, certainly the phenomenon is important enough to merit a change in our ideas about the permeability and multiplicity of our consciousness.

Experience must write upon the brain. It does so in banal ways, as when we learn a new association between, say, a red light and the need to stop. There is work under way on the neurophysiological coding of memory traces in the different systems of the brain. But experience writes larger when there are systematic changes in the environment, since the brain develops to live within one small world of one organism at a time. Changes in experience, above or below the optimal level, can actually change the physiology of the brain.

Remember that our social nature is dependent on our being born immature. Environmental conditions play a greater role in the brain development of human beings than in any other animal. Although it is commonly thought that at birth the neurons begin to make connections and that these connections increase as we age and acquire experience, the opposite appears to be the case. There are many *more* connections in the brain of an infant than in an elderly adult. Development seems to be a matter of "pruning" the original connections rather than making new ones.

The infant babbling utters almost every sound of every known language and later on loses the ability to make those that are not in the language he or she has learned to speak. There is thus a universe of potential sound patterns available to us at birth, but we learn only a few of them. Similarly, the brain may be "set up" at birth to do a myriad of different things, but we only get around to doing a few of them.

The brain, like a muscle, shrinks and grows in response to certain experiences—the neurons actually become larger and smaller with experiences. In a long series of studies at the University of California, Berkeley, Marion Diamond has shown that when rats are deprived of adequate stimulation, their cortexes shrink. She places rats in cages in which their activity is either restricted, or it is close to that of a normal rat in the wild, with "toys" all around and lots of social rat-type interactions. Diamond can find changes in the growth of the nerve dendrites and the numbers of nerve dendrites with these changes in experience. The neurons of the brain thin out with too little stimulation. This developmental process goes on as long as the organism lives and is active. Brain growth can be stimulated in *old* rats when there is new and increased stimulation for as little as one week. The brain is modifiable, and it grows with experience and stimulation.

While overstimulation is commonly associated with stress and other deleterious effects, it also appears to be the case that understimulation can also cause the nervous system to go awry. What happens to health with understimulation, then? In one early study, H. B. Andervont isolated mice into separate cages, some at five weeks and some at twenty weeks of age. Of those who developed cancer, the isolated animals developed mammary tumors earlier than did the mice that were housed eight in a cage. O. Muhlbock also tried to test the effects of crowding and isolation on mammary cancer. At twenty-one days of age, mice were put into one of several conditions: a cage containing fifty animals; another cage partitioned into ten sections containing five animals; a small glass jar containing five animals; and a round pot containing one animal. Each group consisted of ninety to one hundred animals and remained in its assigned environment until the members' natural deaths. In the cage housing fifty animals, 29 percent developed mammary cancer. In the partitioned cage 56 percent developed tumors. The groups of five animals housed in glass jars showed 67 percent incidence. Mice left alone in the round pot seemed to develop the most tumors, but the sample size was too low to be definitive. As in Andervont's study, the isolated animals, the ones receiving suboptimal stimulation, displayed the highest amount of tumor incidence.

Cancer cells are the progeny of normal cells. It does not matter what the cell is; almost any type of specific organ cells—skin, kidney, nerve—can be transformed into cancer cells. Masses of cancer cells (which are called malignant tumors) vary enormously in how much and how fast they grow. Malignant tumors can grow rapidly and explosively, while benign tumors tend to grow very slowly, respecting the boundaries of neighboring healthy tissues.

The fact that a cancer cell is constantly dividing does not distinguish it from normal cells. In mature animals many normal cells are in constant growth and division; they replace the large number of cells that die each day. Cancer cells are less responsive to the normal control devices that cause the cells not to divide. Normal cells seem to be able to recognize when things are getting too crowded inside. It seems to be the extreme deviation from normal stimulation—too far away from our "set point for incoming information"—which causes the problem.

There are other puzzling factors in cancer, some of which may be easier to understand from the viewpoint of the need of the organism for an optimal level of information flow. Human skin contains melanin, a pigment-forming structure, and the amount of melanin varies in different races and individuals. Melanin receives stimulation from solar (ultraviolet) radiation. If the middle range of stimulation were appropriate, then lightly pigmented individuals (light hair, blue eyes, and freckles) would be more susceptible to carcinogenesis via an excess of solar radiation while darkly pigmented individuals would be more susceptible to skin cancer associated with underload.

In light-skinned people, skin cancer occurs most frequently in those areas of the body which are exposed to ultraviolet radiation; those with more pigment sunburn much less readily than do people with light skin and have much less skin cancer. The surprise is that when skin cancer does develop on dark-skinned individuals it is *not* predominantly found on areas of skin exposed to solar radiation. There are reports suggesting that skin cancer can therefore result from too little exposure to ultraviolet solar radiation: Skin cancer in blacks occurs in those areas of the body that are *covered* by clothing.

In one study, white United States war veterans showed a high incidence of cancer on exposed areas of the skin (8.45 percent of all cancer) and black veterans very little (0.6 percent). On the other hand, the percentages for cancers of unexposed skin areas are reversed completely in blacks and whites—0.8 percent in white and 9.78 percent in black veterans. Sixty-one percent of the carcinomas developed in unexposed areas; malignant melanomas occurred most frequently on the sole of the foot.

So there are some intriguing puzzles relating the amount of stimulation we receive (whether from light or social interaction) and the development of cancer. What about our ability to adapt to ever-increasing amounts of information? Could mental factors be important? If so, you might predict that the lower the degree of ability to automatically respond, the less cancer. There is a little evidence on this; not enough to build a house on, but enough to dig a little further.

Herbert Snow observed in 1893 that mentally retarded individuals have a lower cancer rate. He summarized causes of death among the mentally ill and mentally deficient population in England, Wales, Canada, and South Africa and contrasted the rates with those of the general population. Over the period 1865–70, he showed that cancer caused 20 percent of the deaths in the population, but only 8 percent of the deaths among mentally ill and mentally deficient. Of course this could have been due to hundreds of different things; they might have died due to bad food, associated disorders, or lack of exercise.

Jeanne Achterberg recently did perhaps the best controlled study of the different kinds of mental development as they relate to malignancy. With a sample of 3,214 deaths reported by the Texas Department of Mental Health and Mental Retardation over 3½-year periods, she showed that death from cancer in the mentally retarded was only 4 percent of total deaths compared to 18 percent in the general population. This was consistent across age, sex, and race. It did not seem to be only the institutionalization. Average age at death for retarded cancer victims was 43.7 years, 10 years lower than noncancer victims. In general, the lower the IQ, the lower the individual's ability to communicate, help himself and develop satisfactory sensory motor skills, the lower the incidence of cancer.

There is also some Soviet evidence on experiential factors in cancer. In Russian studies in which the central nervous system was stimulated directly by drugs, there is evidence about the importance of the level of activation of the nervous system in cancer development. V. N. Fadeeva in the early fifties examined the influence of different doses of amphetamine on central nervous system stimulation and cancer. Small doses of amphetamine were observed to increase cortical activation, but large doses had a paradoxical effect; they seemed to depress central nervous system activation.

Later studies, also in Russia, examined the differential effects of these high and low doses of amphetamine on the development of cancer. Animals given extremely high doses of amphetamine, caffeine, or strychnine showed an increase in the rate of malignant tumor development while animals given small doses displayed increased cortical activation and a correspondingly lower development of their cancers. In studies of human breast cancer, there are confirming effects. There is association between the use of reserpine, which is a central nervous system (CNS) depressant (a tranquilizing drug) and development of breast cancer.

Augustin de la Peña, in one of the more intriguing hypotheses of recent years, suggests that spontaneous, rapidly spreading cancers are promoted by the information underload (boredom)

experienced by the brain over some relatively prolonged temporal interval. When the information deficit reaches some critical value, the brain sends a nonspecific signal to most somatic structure sites (usually non-CNS structures) indicating the need for novelty or information; carcinogenesis is the body's mode of providing "information-novelty" which is subsequently fed back to the brain and which attempts to rectify the relative information underload signaled by the brain. In the later stages, the development of cancer is also associated with an increase in the disorganization (entropy) of the organismic system.

The increased disorganization is associated with an increase in the amount of information processed from the environment. In the late terminal stages the cancer may also provide information to the CNS in the form of pain by invading or pressing on surrounding tissues which are supplied with nerves, or by leading to pressure on nerves themselves. The pain is then fed back to the brain to help rectify the brain-signaled information deficit. Conversely, chronic information *overload* for the brain is posited to result in a compensatory response by the brain to *decrease* the probability of novelty, i.e. cancer, obtaining in most somatic structure sites.

These are tentative speculations, of course, and do not fully explain the range of factors associated with the disparate family of diseases we call cancer. And yet this point of view is intriguing in that it attempts to bridge brain function and bodily disorders and at least invites investigation of mental factors in carcinogenesis.

So our brain may well try and keep the load of information stable. When there are too many changes and too much information, or when there is too little stimulation and boredom, different kinds of disorder may well result. The brain seems to require a certain degree of latitude in order to control the optimal rate of information inflow and to balance demands with resources.

Several studies of job stress in the United States and Sweden support this view. It is not just high job demands such as noise, heat, physical exertion, and repetitive work that determine the development of cardiovascular disease. However, when high demands are combined with diminished job latitude that restricts the worker from controlling the rate of work or using supportive resources, disease results. For example, preventing a worker from contacting his family during the work day could affect his perception of social support available and thereby decrease his ability to manage work demands. These studies suggest that the lowest degrees of heart disease develop in those workers with medium demands and high latitude to adjust to them.

We hardly suggest that all the studies reviewed above make up an airtight case, but they do support a different way of looking at stress and the role of the brain in managing an optimal information flow as part of its primary job of minding the body. This view also sets the stage for understanding the stress-management resources at the disposal of the brain and why it is that not everyone exposed to stress becomes ill.

CHAPTER FIFTEEN

OF HARDINESS, COHERENCE, AND STABILITY

*L*ife did not start out well for Michael. His mother was sixteen years old, unwed, and lived with her mother and grandmother. She managed to hide her pregnancy from her own mother until the third trimester when she married a nineteen-year-old boy. The child's biological father was very much against the marriage. The mother did not receive any medical attention until the seventh month of pregnancy, and Michael was born prematurely and weighed only four pounds ten ounces. Michael spent the first three weeks of his life in an army hospital. At two, Michael's adoptive father was sent with the army to Korea, where he remained for two years. At age eight, Michael's parents divorced and his mother left, leaving him with his father and three younger siblings.

Early life was also not easy for Kay. She was born of seventeen-year-old unmarried parents. They had both been asked to leave school because of the pregnancy, and the father was without a job. Kay's mother was sent by the Family Court to a Salvation Army Home to have her baby; placing her for adoption was considered but rejected, and the parents were eventually married when Kay was six months old despite objections from their parents. Kay's parents later separated.

Mary got off to a rough start as well. Her mother's pregnancy occurred after many unsuccessful attempts to conceive and a previous miscarriage. Her mother was very much overweight and had various minor medical problems during pregnancy. She was hospitalized three times for severe false labor and eventually was in labor for more than twenty hours. During childhood her parents experienced financial difficulties, and her mother found it necessary to work outside the home for short periods. Between Mary's fifth and tenth birthdays, her mother had several major illnesses, surgeries, and two hospitalizations for "unbearable tension," nervousness, annoyance with her children, and fears that she might harm them.

Despite their many difficulties and disadvantages in early life, Michael, Kay, and Mary grew up to be healthy, well-adjusted, successful adults. Michael ranked at the top of his class and received a college scholarship. He was described as confident, persistent, self-assured, dependable, and realistic. He was liked by his peers.

Kay was an affectionate, healthy, robust and alert baby. As a child she was described as agreeable, relaxed, and mentally normal with above-average grades in school. As an adult she planned to go into the entertainment field and marry. She was characterized as poised, sociable, self-assured, but respectful and accepting of others. While not overly ambitious, she did make quite good use of the abilities she had.

Mary at age eighteen described herself this way: "If I say how I am it sounds like bragging—I have a good personality and people like me . . . I don't like it when people think they can run my own life—I like to be my own judge. I know right from wrong, but I feel I have a lot more to learn and go through. Generally, I hope I can make it—I hope." She planned to enroll in college and was keeping her future career goals open. She was described as being high in self-esteem, outgoing, persistent, and concerned with others as well as willing to open herself up to new possibilities after initial hesitancies.

What is the source of their strength and resilience?

Michael, Kay, and Mary were three people observed in a landmark twenty-year study of children growing up on Kauai, in Hawaii. They were part of a large study of nearly seven hundred children followed from a few months before their birth into their early twenties. They were assessed an intervals with a battery of interviews, examinations, questionnaires, and review of health records.

All of these children came from poor families and were raised by mothers who had not graduated from high school and by fathers who were semiskilled or unskilled laborers. They came of age in the years 1955 to 1979—a time of unprecedented social change. They had to deal with the influx of many newcomers from the U.S. mainland during the long war in Southeast Asia and later with the burgeoning of tourism. They witnessed the assassination of one president and the resignation of another. They were the first generation to deal with the invasion of the home by television. They faced unprecedented choices since they had access to contraceptive pills and mind-altering drugs.

By all standards these children were at high risk: born and raised in chronic poverty, exposed to higher-than-average rates of premature birth and perinatal stress, and reared by mothers with little formal education. In combination, these biological and social stressors took their toll, resulting in the development of serious learning and behavior problems in childhood and adolescence.

Yet some survived and even thrived in the face of these stresses. They somehow managed to develop into competent, confident, autonomous adults who "worked well, played well, loved well, and expected well." What distinguished the one in ten who were "resilient"? What was different about their behavior and their caregiving environment that protected them from the serious coping problems which developed in their peers?

In their book *Vulnerable, But Invincible,* Emmy Werner and Ruth Smith detail their remarkable study of seventy-two resilient children. Their findings help identify some of the factors which relate to this kind of resilience. Their mothers reported that the children were active and "socially responsive" even when they were infants, and other observers reported they had positive social orientations when young children. Their interests, in childhood and in adolescence, weren't determined by their sex. They seemed to have a strong concept of themselves and could follow their interests where they led. According to the study, they had

a more positive self-concept, and a more nurturant, responsible, and achievement-oriented attitude toward life than peers who developed serious coping problems. . . . At the threshold of adulthood, the resilient men and women had developed a sense of coherence in their lives and were able to draw on a number of informal sources of support. They also expressed a desire to "improve themselves," i.e., toward continued psychological growth.

What were the key factors in the early environment that appeared to contribute to the resiliency and stress resistance of these high-risk children?

These families were poor by material standards, but a characteristically strong bond was forged between the infant and the primary caretaker during the first year of life. The physical robustness of the resilient children, their high activity level, and their social responsiveness were recognized by the caregivers and elicited a great deal of attention. There was little prolonged separation of the infants from their mothers and no prolonged bond disruption during the first year of life. The strong attachment that resulted appears to have been a secure base for the development of advanced self-help skills and autonomy noted among these children in their second year of life.

Though many of their mothers worked for extended periods and were major contributors to family subsistence, the children had support from alternative caretakers, such as grandmothers or older sisters, to whom they became attached.

Many resilient children grew up in multiage households that included members of the grandparent generation. As older siblings departed from the household, the resilient girls took responsibility for the care of younger siblings. The employment of their mothers and the need for sibling caretaking seems to have contributed to a greater autonomy and sense of responsibility in the resilient girls, especially in households were the father was dead or otherwise absent. Their competence was enhanced by a strong bond between the daughter and the other females in the family—sometimes across three generations.

Resilient boys, in turn, were often first-born sons, lived in smaller families, and did not have to share their parents' attention with many additional children in the first decade of life. There were some males in their family who could serve as models for identification (fathers, older brothers, or uncles). There was a structure and rules in the household, but space to explore in and less physical crowding. Last, but not least, there was an informal, multiage network of kin, peers, and elders who shared similar values and beliefs, and from whom the resilient youth sought counsel and support in times of crises and major role transitions.

This study, and others of children of schizophrenic parents or children surviving war, abuse, and adversity, give testimony to the enormous self-righting tendencies of the human organism. These investigations are beginning to reshape our thinking about stress and the resistance to disease. The attitude of current "stress = disease" workers is unfortunately like that of their germ-oriented predecessors in medicine: In both cases the external agents are somehow supposed to act on a defenseless, mindless organism.

Like the deadly germs of earlier centuries, stress has become the feared plague of the twentieth century. Stressors abound. Job pressures, deadlines, being hired, being fired, marital discord, death of loved ones, shoelaces that break, cars that don't work, traffic that won't move, and on and on. No one can escape.

Such stressful life events, whether major trauma or minor hassles, take their toll. Wear us down. Make us more vulnerable to all disorders from cancer to heart attacks, infections to depression. However, the simple equation—stressor "in" (whether it be psychological trauma or microbes) equals disease "out"— doesn't really work. It doesn't help us understand why most people exposed to stressors don't become ill. Or why two people confronting the same stressor react so differently, one breaking down and the other seeming to thrive.

The popular view, supported by many researchers, therapists, and certainly the media, is that stress kills: "Watch out for stressors and try to avoid them at all costs." But this pessimistic view of people as passive victims of stress doesn't really make sense. If we really followed this advice and tried to avoid stressors no one would ever marry, have children, take a job, get divorced, or invent anything at all.

Most people need change and challenge. They seek out novelty and stimulation. Many come through stressful experiences not with illness but with better strength and health. For many people disease is not inevitable in the face of difficulty.

Even though the relationship between events such as moving from one city to another and subsequent disease is important, the correlations are modest and may hide more than they reveal. If you try to predict who will become ill based on a tally of major life events, you are likely to be correct only about 15 percent of the time. This means that there is a large group of people who are not exposed to high stress yet become ill. But more interesting, perhaps, are the people who survive and remain healthy in the face of changes and challenges in their lives.

We do not have to consider ourselves as somehow without resources in the face of the awesome and ever-changing modern world. It has begun to be recognized that a person in the face of all this instability, wild change, and tumult is not powerless: He or she already *has a brain* that possesses the evolved network of 500 million years of nerve circuits that can deal with the continual changes.

The most important question, once again, is not about alleviating sickness, but about maintaining health; not why people break down under stress, but how it is that anyone maintains health given all the stressors that everyone must encounter in the normal course of living.

The traditional view holds that stressors, physical or psychological, almost automatically trigger the flight-or-fight reaction in the body. This reaction, if frequent, severe, and persistent, can produce a variety of symptoms like headache, insomnia, gastrointestinal distress, and back pain. It also leaves one vulnerable to disease agents. Then, depending upon biological constitution and exposure, one person may develop heart disease, another cancer, yet another a peptic ulcer.

But this chain of events from stressor to illness is not inevitable. When confronted with a stressor, some people seem to be able to cope with it without becoming anxious and aroused in a harmful way. Some people appraise the potential stressor in such a way as to avoid stress. The charging lion may elicit a very difference reaction in you than in the experienced animal trainer. Other people are able to take action in the face of a stressor which minimizes or eliminates the threat.

What are the characteristics of these stress-resistant people? Suzanne Kobasa, a social psychologist, and her colleagues identified the elements of psychological hardiness. She initially studied a group of middle- and upper-level business executives at Illinois Bell Telephone Company, a division of AT&T, at the time the company was preparing for divestiture—one of the largest corporate reorganizations in history. It was a time of great stress and uncertainty.

Nearly seven hundred executives were asked about the type and frequency of certain stressful life changes as well as illnesses they had experienced in the previous three years. A subsample of two hundred was then selected from those who had scored high on the stress scale. About half of them did experience high levels of illness, but the other half remained healthy in the face of stress.

What distinguished the high stress/high illness executives from the high stress/low illness ones? They were similar in terms of income, job status, educational levels, age, ethnic background, and religious identification and practice. But they were very different in terms of their attitudes about themselves, their jobs, and the people around them.

The psychological hardiness of the high stress/low illness executives was characterized by a strong *commitment* to self, work, family, and other important values, a sense of *control* over one's life, and the ability to see change in one's life as a *challenge* rather than a threat.

These hardy people accepted that change, rather than stability, was the norm in life and tended to welcome it as an opportunity for growth. They sought novelty, tolerated ambiguity, and demonstrated a cognitive flexibility and strong sense of purpose in approaching life's problems. They would agree with statements like: "I would be willing to sacrifice financial stability in my work if something really challenging came along" or "I often wake up eager to start on the day's projects" or "Trying my best at work makes a difference."

In contrast, the high stress/high illness executives were low in hardiness, displaying a strong sense of alienation and powerlessness. They were threatened by change and suffered in the face of uncertainty. Low-hardiness people would tend to agree with statements like: "Trusting in fate is sometimes all I can do" or "Getting close to people puts me at risk of being obligated to them" or "It bothers me when I have to deviate from the routine or schedule I have set for myself." In one of our symposia, Suzanne Kobasa said that it is difficult to fathom what they are really like. She describes one encounter:

> "I'm thinking of making a major change; I'm thinking of leaving the phone company and going to this little electronics company that's a much more risky operation, and I figure if what you're going to do is free, I'll come and get the advice. Maybe it'll be helpful." This man's protocol showed high stress and high illness. He was only in his thirties, but he had hypertension, peptic ulcer, and migraine headaches: many symptoms as well as diseases.

What stands out from his personality questionnaire is alienation, not only from himself but also from other people. He also shows some low control, but the main factor is the alienation, the lack of commitment that is striking.

He arrives forty-five minutes late, trenchcoat flying behind him, papers under his arm. Then he makes a beeline for my secretary's desk and begins calling people. He's got to call many people to let them know where he's going to be in the next forty-five minutes, while I'm in my office waiting, hearing all these phone calls. He comes in and I've prepared what's going to be a fairly difficult conversation with him about his alienation from other people, but it's difficult to do that because the phone keeps ringing and every time it does he jumps up because he's convinced it's for him and he can't talk in my office so he has to run out to the secretary's office. This happens three times and we're not getting anywhere.

He says to me, "Look, I really need to take all these calls, they're very crucial. But you may have something here. So why don't you talk into my tape recorder?" So he pulls out a tape recorder, puts it on my desk and says, "I'll listen to it at night when I have a chance."

Suzanne Kobasa and Salvatore Maadi also describe the hardy:

Bill B. is the kind of person who has an immediately reassuring effect on those around him. At fifty-five years of age, he has a twinkle in his eye and an easy, relaxed manner. He seems to have all the time in the world as he asks the interviewer what the research is about and how it is done. All the details seem interesting to him. . . .

When he begins to describe his work at the phone company, the curiosity he has for what he does not know shades over into zest for the familiar. He embellishes his descriptions all the while making his role in planning commercial telephone services come alive. Although he has a clear sense of the importance of broader social issues concerning his work, and certainly feels that his role requires innovative planning, it is the moment-to-moment activities of the day that intrigue him the most. He claims to learn fairly continuously, even when the task appears at first to be routine.

When asked his views about the company reorganization, he expresses a clear sense of the magnitude of the changes in the offing. But he shows no signs of the panic we saw in other subjects. He is not more certain than they are about what the changes will mean for him specifically. But he is so involved and interested in the evolutionary process going on that he almost welcomes it. Whatever his new role turns out to be, he is sure he will find a way to make it meaningful and worthwhile. He recognizes the hard work and possible frustrations involved in the company's reorganization, but he treats it as all in a day's work. He looks forward to rolling up his sleeves, working hard and learning new things—he is involved with the company and wants to help with its reorganization.

Bill's wife died seven years ago in an accident while they were on vacation. He can still evoke the pain and shock of that unfortunate event. Her death depressed him for more than a year, though he showed few signs of guilt. He missed her more than he felt guilty. . . . Since his wife's death, Bill has lived alone. Although this was difficult at first, he has long since developed a satisfying routine. When he wants company, he invites friends for a meal he enjoys cooking or visits his children or grandchildren. Often, however, he spends time alone, reading or building furniture, and does not feel lonely. . . . He enjoys satisfying social interactions yet is not bored when alone. Even when he relaxes, he finds much in himself and the passing scene that is of interest.

Reflecting on the early part of his married life, Bill recounted some fortunate and unfortunate events—his son's hernia operation, the deaths of his grandparents, a fire in the family home. Although he discusses these events vividly, he experiences them as part of life, as the things that helped make him the person he is now. He sees these negative and positive events in balance, the regrets mitigated by the satisfactions. . . .

Bill remains basically quite healthy. Signs of mental and physical strain are mild to nonexistent. Despite the relatively high number of symptoms typical of people in his age category, Bill has avoided any serious illnesses.

Hardy personalities tend to view and cope with life's problems quite differently than others—when a person low in hardiness loses his job he is more likely to view it as a catastrophe which confirms his own sense of worthlessness. A hardy sort is likely to see the job loss as within the range of expected risks when she took it. She might even view the job loss as an opportunity to seek out new employment better suited to her capabilities.

These differences in appraisal can result in enormous differences in how people respond to potentially stressful events. Hardy people transform problems into opportunities and thereby do not elicit a stress response in the first place. Unhardies (softies?) distract themselves from the problem with drugs, television, or social interaction. This kind of "avoidance coping" can be useful when the problem is insoluble, but when something can be done to alter the stressor and is not, the source of stress remains and is more likely to mobilize a chronic stress reaction with illness as a consequence. The findings correlating hardiness with health in the face of stress were confirmed in a prospective study. Over 250 business managers were surveyed three times over a two-year period. Pinpointing the hardiness characteristics of challenge, commitment, and control helped predict which of the stressed executives would get ill and which would remain well. The hardy executives were only one-half as likely to get sick as less hardy people confronting similar stressors.

The findings also apply to other professional groups (lawyers and army officers) as well as women visiting their gynecologists' offices. In the study of army officers a curious finding emerged. The commitment and control elements of hardiness appeared to help protect the officer faced with high levels of life stress, but those officers who demonstrated a challenge orientation were more prone to become ill.

This finding prompts us to consider the match between the person and his environment, his resources and the demands, as perhaps more important than the personality characteristics alone. In *The Great Santini*, Robert Duvall plays a test pilot of the mid-fifties, just after the Korean War. The Great Santini gets into scrapes, has disciplinary problems himself and with his children, and puts strain on his marriage. He dies in a plane crash on a training mission. As he describes himself, he is "a war hero without a war," a man needing challenge and conflict, but finding too little. Similarly, in the post-Vietnam army there was little room for those seeking novelty or challenge. When a person's challenge orientation is not matched by the opportunities for it, more illness can result. As we have seen, people need to find the right set point for stimulation and challenge in their lives.

Hardiness is not the only thing that helps protect people from stress. A strong inherited constitution, exercise, and social support can also help. Kobasa and her colleagues examined the family histories of the Illinois Bell executives for indications of increased risk of disorders likely to have a strong genetic contribution, such as cancer, heart disease, and rheumatoid arthritis. Not surprisingly, they found the individuals with a stronger family history of disease were more likely to become ill. However, biology is not destiny. The hardy remained healthier in the face of stress than the less hardy, even if the hardy person had a stronger family history of disease.

Hardy executives also seemed to take better advantage of social support to protect their health. Curiously, though, executives low in hardiness appeared to be hurt by strong emotional support from their family. Consider an executive who feels helpless, alienated, and threatened at work. He goes home and finds a warm, supportive wife and family. They comfort him as best as they can but do little to help him solve the specific problems he faces at work. In fact, instead of trying to engage and solve the problems at work, the executive might find it tempting to retreat to the safe haven of home. The result is greater reported illness among the stressed executives with low hardiness and strong family support.

However, executives, whether hardy or not, who received strong support from their bosses were less likely to become ill. This suggests that certain types of social support may be needed to help deal with certain types of problems. When the source of stress is work-related changes, support from one's boss appears to be most helpful and protective.

Hardiness, exercise, and social support combined to protect the health of executives under stress. The likelihood of illness developing in stressed executives with none of these resistance resources was 93 percent, 72 percent in those with one resource, 58 percent in those with two, and dropping to less than 8 percent in those who were hardy, exercised, and had good social support.

Can one learn to become hardier? From their interviews with hardy executives and others Kobasa and Maadi identified characteristics of early childhood experiences which seem to foster the development of hardiness. Commitment seems to emerge from strong parental encouragement and acceptance. Control is cultivated in children successfully encountering a variety of tasks which are neither too simple nor too difficult.

And a challenge orientation is more likely to develop when the child is faced with a changing environment which is construed as richness rather than chaos. These features also appear to foster hardiness in adults. A work environment which encourages self-mastery of a variety of tasks and is accompanied by strong encouragement by peers and superiors is more likely to assist in the development of hardiness.

Maadi and Kobasa have also developed "hardiness induction

groups," which are small group sessions designed specifically to encourage a sense of commitment, control, and challenge. Group members are taught how to focus on their bodies and mental sensations in response to stressful situations. They are encouraged to ask themselves questions like "What's keeping me from feeling terrific today?" This focusing increases their sense of control over stress.

People are also encouraged to think about a recent stressful episode and imagine three ways it might have been worse and three ways it could have gone better. In addition, group members are given ideas of what to do when they come face to face with a stressor they cannot avoid or control, like the death of a spouse or a serious illness. They are encouraged to refocus on another area of their lives in which they can master a new challenge and restore their sense of control and competence. They might learn a new skill like swimming or offer their services in tutoring.

The preliminary result of this hardiness training is encouraging. A group of eight high-stress, hypertensive executives attended eight weekly group sessions. At the end, not only were their hardiness scores higher, but they reported fewer symptoms of psychological distress and their blood pressures were lower when compared to an untreated control group.

Sometimes active coping through direct problem solving is not possible even for the hardiest. Some events cannot be avoided or changed by confronting them directly. The mind may become flooded with anxious thoughts. Memories or anticipations of threatening situations intrude into consciousness. Fortunately, the brain evolved with mechanisms to deal with anxiety and psychic discomfort, mechanisms that clear the deck and make possible other thoughts and actions.

One such mechanism is denial, the mental operation by which thoughts, feelings, acts, threats, or demands are minimized or negated. Unfortunately, denial has gotten bad press, viewed as a negative defense mechanism which leads to pathology. People must face reality, "get in touch with their feelings," and be honest about them. Illusion, self-deception, and denial are unhealthy and must be rooted out, perhaps in therapy. Yet this traditional view is not consistent with some of the newer information about how the brain works. Sometimes we need our illusions.

Psychologist Richard Lazarus argues that illusion has positive value in a person's psychological economy:

The fabric of our lives is woven in part from illusions and unexamined beliefs. There is, for example, the collective illusion that our society is free, moral, and just, which, of course, isn't always true. Then there are the countless idiosyncratic beliefs people hold about themselves and the world in which they live—for example, that we are better than average, or doomed to fail, or that the world is a benign conspiracy, or that is rigged against us. Many such beliefs are passed down from parent to child and never challenged. Despite the fixity with which people hold such beliefs, they have little or no basis in reality. One's person's beliefs are another's delusions. In effect, we pilot our lives in part by illusions and by self-deceptions that give meaning and substance to life.

As we have seen, the brain works by constructing a reality from a narrow trickle of information received, reduced and filtered through the senses. These constructed beliefs, many based on denial and illusion, have adaptive value.

It should not come as a surprise that the brain has adaptive mechanisms to block or attenuate painful stimuli, whether due to physical injury or psychological trauma. The elaborate intrinsic pain relief system, in part mediated by endorphins, has evolved to be able to block transmission of pain stimuli. This system appears to be turned on during acutely stressful situations when the organism must prepare to flee or fight. Numbing pain when being attacked by a charging wild animal would allow the organism to ignore physical trauma and handle the immediate threat.

Analogously, the brain has developed certain adaptive mechanisms like denial, which can help block perception of certain threatening information when attending to it will only arouse unnecessary anxiety and contribute little to changing the situation. Therefore, whether denial is healthy or not depends on the circumstances and outcome.

There are situations in which denial can interfere with necessary actions and thereby undermine health. The diabetic who needs to carefully regulate insulin dosages, the patient with kidney disease who needs to undergo dialysis, or the woman who discovers a breast lump all need to pay attention to information about their health in order to take actions to preserve it. Denying a breast lump can lead to delays in treatment for breast cancer. The patient with chest pain who does push-ups or runs up and down stairs to prove he is not having a heart attack clearly illustrates the danger of unhealthy denial.

A study of asthmatics compared those patients who responded to symptoms with vigilance and those who tended to disregard them. At the first sign of an asthmatic attack the vigilant patients became alert and fearful, while the others denied the seriousness of the symptoms, expecting that the attack would not occur. The high-fear, vigilant patients were far less likely to be hospitalized for their asthma in a six-month period than the asthmatics who coped with denial. In this situation, the vigilance was helpful, presumably because it allowed the patients to take some corrective action to avert a more severe asthmatic attack.

But denial can be helpful. Frances Cohen and Richard Lazarus studied sixty-one patients about to undergo elective surgery for conditions like hernia and gall bladder disease. The patients were asked about how much they knew or wanted to know about the disease, the operation, and so on. Two basic coping strategies were vigilance and avoidance.

The avoiders denied the emotional or threatening aspects of the surgery and were not interested in thinking about or listening to anything that was related to their illness or surgery. They would say things like: "All I know is that I have a hernia. I just took it for granted. It doesn't disturb me one bit. I have not thought at all about it."

In contrast, the vigilant were quite alert to the emotional and threatening aspects of the upcoming medical event. They attempted to cope by trying to control every detail of the situation and were aroused to every danger. One vigilant patient commented after a detailed description of the operation: "I have all the facts, my will is prepared. It is major surgery. It's a body opening. You're put out, you could be put out too deep, your heart could quit, you can have a shock. I go not in lightly."

When compared, the avoiders seemed to fare better in the post-surgical recovery period than the vigilant. The avoiders were discharged from the hospital sooner, had fewer minor complications (nausea, headache, fever, infection), required less pain medication, and showed less distress. Some of the improved outcome may be due to the different way the vigilant are treated by the doctor. Since they are more likely to notice and report symptoms after the operation, the doctor is perhaps more likely to conclude that the patient is not ready to go home. However, extreme vigilance in this pre- and postsurgical setting may be counterproductive since it mobilizes the brain and triggers a stress reaction when there is little the patient can actually do to influence the outcome.

There are other situations in which denial may be healthy. Immediately following an acute crisis or catastrophic illness, such as a spinal cord injury or a severe burn, the victim may be able to buy some time by denying the implications of his trauma. Denying the severity of an incapacitating disease may be a helpful first step in coping with it. A temporary disavowal of reality helps a person get through the devastating early period of loss and threat when there is in truth little he can do. Later the person can face the facts at a gradual, more manageable pace and mobilize other means of coping.

Richard Lazarus observed:

> Illusion can sometimes allow hope, which is healthy. The critical determinant is whether you're denying facts or the implications. Implications are ambiguous. Let's say I get a biopsy that says I have a malignant tumor. I can face the facts, decide this is a terrible illness, that I'm in trouble, will die very soon, and so give up hope. Or I can face the fact that this is a serious illness, but acknowledge the ambiguity; people sometimes recover; it's curable. I've got to be treated, but I don't have to give up.

Flexibility appears to be central to successful coping—the wisdom to know when to use denial and when other more active means of coping are more useful. Consider a person who has had a heart attack. At different stages in the illness different means of coping would be adaptive. At the onset of chest pain, denial is dangerous. Action, namely getting immediate medical assistance, is required.

However, once in the hospital or once under medical care some denial and avoidance may be adaptive. Several studies of patients in an intensive care unit following a heart attack have found that survival is better among those who minimized the seriousness of their illnesses and remained calm than with patients who worried and were hypervigilant. Following discharge from the hospital, a different balance of denial and vigilance is most useful. Those patients with excessive denial of their disease are less likely to take their medications, follow an appropriate diet or exercise program, and recovery may be impeded.

On the other hand, those who remain hypervigilant may be

more prone to develop "cardiac neurosis" in which the patient fears a return to normal life lest it provoke a recurrent heart attack. Hence, they may be slower to go back to work, resume sexual activity, and otherwise function normally.

From the viewpoint of the brain and body, arousal, fear, and vigilance are useful only in so far as they alert the brain to take corrective action to ameliorate the threat and instability. When there is nothing that can be done to aid survival, then denying or ignoring the threat protects the stability and health of the person. And, importantly, it leaves room for hope.

In informal discussions, physicians often describe some of their patients as having "lost the will to live" or "having given up hope," somehow suggesting that hope is vital to survival. Yet hope is virtually ignored as a subject of medical research.

Hope represents a special type of positive expectation. Unlike denial, which involves a negation of reality, hope is an active way of coping with threatening situations by focusing on the positive. No matter how dark or grim a situation may appear, certain people seem to be able to extract the positive aspects and concentrate on them. They fill their minds with hopeful scenarios, stories with happy endings, or lucky outcomes.

Hope is not always easy, as David Sobel found out:

> I was recently confronted with a highly stressful situation, a life-threatening illness in a family member. I recall watching my mind struggle between hope and despair. Despair was easy, but hope required continual effort. I think this is because hope implies uncertainty about the future and the brain finds it difficult to maintain a state of uncertainty. Despair at least offers the troubled mind certainty and stability. One may think the outcome is catastrophic, but at least one has certainty and stability in this view.

Nevertheless, difficult though it may be to maintain hope, it appears that hope fosters health. Faced with a threat, say the diagnosis of cancer, one person may focus on the negative: "getting cancer means death," "treatments are useless," "ninety percent of patients are dead in five years." Others may be able to mobilize more hopeful thoughts: "many people have been cured of cancer," "my doctors will do everything possible to help my recovery," "one in ten people survive for longer than five years with this type of cancer, and I could be one of those survivors."

On the other hand, losing hope and becoming helpless has the opposite effect. When a person or animal discovers that it has no control over events that affect it, the result can be helplessness, learning that one's actions do not lead to one's goals. There is a fair amount of research, both animal and human, on the phenomenon of learned helplessness. The basic experiment uses three groups: one group learns that actions can lead to a desired outcome—avoiding something aversive; a second group experiences the same stress as first group, but the members' actions do not avoid the unpleasantness; a third group receives no previous learning experiences. Later, all three groups are tested on a new task.

In one study, a group of dogs in a restraining hammock were trained to turn off shock by pressing a panel with their noses. The second group received shocks just like their partners in the first group, but without any means of control. A third group was placed in hammocks but received no shocks. Twenty-four hours later, all three groups received avoidance training. The first and third group performed well and learned to jump over a barrier to avoid shock. The second group was slower to respond, and six of the eight dogs in this group failed to escape.

It was not the shock itself, but inability to control it that caused the "helpless" failure to escape. Similar responses have been found in cats, fish, rats, and people. Martin Seligman, the innovator of this theory, describes how learned helplessness can lead to depression:

> When a traumatic event first occurs, it causes a heightened state of emotionality that can loosely be called fear. This state continues until one of two things happens: if the subject learns that he can control the trauma, fear is reduced and may disappear altogether; or if the subject finally learns he cannot control the trauma, fear will decrease and be replaced with depression.

If depression, or at least depression developed mainly in reaction to external events, really is learned helplessness, this is important. Considering Seligman's dogs who failed to escape shock: Perhaps experiences of successful escape would teach them that they were not helpless. So Seligman put long leashes on these dogs and dragged them over the barrier, *forcing* them to escape. After twenty-five to two hundred draggings, each dog began to initiate its own response and thereafter never failed to escape. The experience of control can reverse the learning of helplessness.

One can also learn to be hopeful even when one is helpless. Even if one can't control the outcome, as with many serious accidents or illnesses, one can still be hopeful that somehow, from somewhere, help will come, and the situation will change for the better.

But do hope and the belief that things will get better, or that one can make them better, actually make a difference in recovery? What determines whether someone mobilizes hope or despair? Not much is known scientifically about the effects of hope, but there are hints that hope itself may be a powerful force in recovery; new research is beginning to elucidate the physiology of hope and positive expectation.

In some early research A. Schmale and H. Iker looked at whether patients' attitudes of hopefulness or hopelessness could predict cervical cancer. They interviewed sixty-eight women who had come to the hospital for a cervical biopsy to evaluate abnormal pap smear results that contained cells suspicious for cervical cancer. The researchers interviewed the women before anyone knew the results of the biopsies and predicted which women would be more likely to have cancer based on their degree of hopelessness.

Of the sixty-eight women, twenty-eight had cancer and forty did not. The researchers were able to correctly predict 68 percent of the cancer patients based on their hopeless attitudes and 77 percent of the cancer-free women based on their hopefulness. The hopeful patients were clearly less likely to be harboring cancer at the time of the interviews. While it is tempting to assume that the hopeful attitude somehow protected these women from cancer, it is also possible that the hopeless feelings expressed by the cancer victims were the result of the cancer process itself.

The words we use can reflect our degree of hope and may predict those more likely to have cancer. Donald Spence and his colleagues analyzed interviews with sixty-two women before the biopsy results for cervical cancer were known. They looked for certain key words such as *dark, disgusting, difficulty, conflict, cancer,* and *tense,* which suggested a mental state of hopelessness, and other marker words such as *desire, eager, expect, longing, wish,* and *yearn,* which reflected a more hopeful attitude. Again, the more hopeless women were more likely to have a positive biopsy result showing cervical cancer.

What role might hope play in healing and recovery from illness? Take, for example, a group of patients entering the hospital for surgical repair of a detached retina. R. C. Mason and his colleagues surveyed the patients before the operation regarding their trust in the surgeon, optimism about the result, and confidence in their ability to cope with the outcome, whether good or bad. The surgeons, without knowledge of the patients' responses, were then asked to independently rate the speed of healing of the retina following surgery. The degree of hope, trust, and acceptance correlated very highly with the speed of healing.

How are attitudes of hope and positive expectation reflected in brain and body chemistry? New research is just beginning to investigate the correlations between one's thoughts and expectations and one's physiology. The results support the surprising view that our expectations may have more to do with our reaction to stress than the objectively stressful experience itself.

Consider the stressful situation of having to go on a strenuous long march. The performance of the march itself as well as the degree of physiological and psychological stress is determined more by what's in the head than what's in the feet.

Psychologist Shlomo Bresnitz studied the effects of expectation and hope on Israeli soldiers required to go on a long march. The soldiers were divided into four groups and were separated so they could not communicate with each other. All the soldiers marched forty kilometers (about twenty-five miles) over the same terrain on the same day carrying heavy packs.

The soldiers in the first group were told by their officers the exact distance they were expected to go and kept fully informed throughout the march about how far they had traveled. The second group was only told "this is the long march you heard about." They were not told how long it was and were given no information about how far they had traveled. In the third group the soldiers were initially told they had to march thirty kilometers, but then at the last moment were told they had to go another ten. The soldiers in the fourth group were told at first they had to march sixty kilometers but were stopped at forty.

So all these groups actually marched the same distance but with different thoughts in their heads.

The effects of the march were measured in terms of morale,

performance (including how many dropped out during the march), and in changes in serum cortisol and prolactin, two hormones whose levels are thought to rise as stress increases.

The soldiers who were given the realistic information and who were kept fully informed on how far they had to go performed the best with the least evidence of stress. These men demonstrated the highest degree of hopefulness based on clear information of what was expected. The light at the end of the tunnel helped them on.

The group that was given no information at all fared the worst. When these men were asked to estimate how far they had gone some thought it was a short distance, others very long. Interestingly their subjective estimates of distance correlated better with serum cortisol levels than did the actual distance traveled. The stress of the difficult march was more in the brain than in the foot.

Of the groups who were given false information, those who thought they were going thirty kilometers were discouraged when told they had to go ten kilometers farther but nevertheless finished the march. However, those that were told they had to go sixty kilometers at the outset were completely demoralized. Many of them dropped out after only ten. Of those that continued on, by the time they heard that they only had to go forty kilometers, they were so exhausted and hopeless that it didn't matter much.

Beliefs and expectations are powerful. Certain positive attitudes, particularly perceptions about one's own health and capabilities, appear to be correlated with better health. Consider the series of experiments conducted by Ann O'Leary, Kate Lorig, and their colleagues at the Stanford Arthritis Center. The project began innocently enough. An arthritis self-management course was designed to help patients with arthritis cope better with the pain, disability, fear, and depression often associated with the disease. The program consisted of six weekly two-hour sessions attended by patients and their families and led by instructors, many of whom had arthritis themselves. They learned basic information about the pathophysiology and treatment of arthritis, strengthening and endurance exercises, relaxation techniques, joint protection, nutrition, and the interrelationship of stress, pain, and depression.

The results were impressive. Compared to a control group

(who had to wait four months before beginning the course), the participants demonstrated significantly greater knowledge, self-management behavior, and less pain. But why? The usual assumption would be that knowledge increased, behavior changed (practice of therapeutic exercises) and reduced pain was the result. The problem was that the data did not support this conclusion.

The people who improved were not necessarily the ones who knew more about arthritis or engaged in therapeutic exercise. What did predict those who would improve? Careful interviews with class participants suggested that those who improved had a positive outlook and felt a sense of control regarding their arthritis. Those who failed to improve, even if they exercised, felt "there was nothing they could do about their arthritis."

The key difference appeared to be the person's perception of his or her own ability to control or change the arthritis symptoms. This quality, which has been termed "self-efficacy," reflects a person's own judgment and conviction that he or she can perform a specific action. Notice that the critical feature here is the person's belief in his or her capacity, not what skills or capacities the person actually has.

With regard to the improvement in arthritis symptoms, the best predictor was how likely the person *thought* he or she would be to improve. The arthritis self-management classes were accordingly reorganized to maximize this sense of self-efficacy. The participants were encouraged to set their own goals, breaking them down in very small achievable steps to insure success. Feeling confident that one is able to walk up two steps may be more helpful than being able to walk up a whole flight but thinking oneself incapable of doing so. Successfully reaching a goal appears to be critical in fostering a better sense of control. Modeling successful coping, encouraging reinforcement, and providing skills to manage anxiety and reinterpret physical symptoms also contribute to self-efficacy.

Participants in the self-management program experienced a 28 percent reduction in pain, a 20 percent decrease in swollen joints, a 14 percent decrease in disability, an 18 percent decrease in depression, and a 20 percent increase in perceived self-efficacy. This time the improvements in symptoms were significantly correlated with perceived self-efficacy.

Other studies have shown that perceived self-efficacy is useful in understanding relapse in smoking cessation programs, pain management, eating disorders, cardiac rehabilitation, and adherence to medical regimens. Albert Bandura and his colleagues documented physiological changes related to changes in "self-efficacy." They studied twelve women with a spider phobia and measured catecholamine secretion, chemical substances released in response to stress.

The level of catecholamine secretion was related to the women's perception of how well they thought they could cope with different tasks involving a spider (looking at a spider, putting a hand in a bowl with a spider, and allowing a spider to crawl on a hand). The higher the perceived capability to deal with the stressful encounter, the less stress and the less catecholamine secretion. When Bandura strengthened the women's sense of self-efficacy with regard to the tasks which aroused the phobic reactions, catecholamine secretion also dropped.

The kinds of psychological processes we have discussed are startlingly important for health. We live our lives within our own small world, bounded by our own beliefs, beliefs that explain the world to us and allow us to act on events, beliefs that mobilize the body and allow us to operate consistently and coherently.

And the health consequences? It is hard to be quantitative about this, but consider this study. If you wanted to predict how likely a person would be to become ill, what would you do? You might review the person's medical history, perform extensive laboratory tests, or perhaps ask for a doctor's assessment of health. Alternatively, you might just ask the person how he viewed his own health.

As it turns out, one of the best predictors of future health is self-rated health. You ask a person: How would you rate your health overall (poor, fair, good, excellent)? Surprisingly, this simple question better predicts a person's health status than objective assessments made by his or her doctor. People who tend to rate their health poorly die earlier and have more disease than their counterparts who view themselves as healthy. Even people with objective disease seem to do better when they believe themselves to be healthy than when they believe themselves to be weak.

In Manitoba, Canada, over thirty-five hundred senior citizens were asked at the outset of a seven-year study, "For your age would you say, in general, your health is excellent, good, fair, poor, or bad?" In addition, their objective health status was determined by reports from their physicians on medical problems and how often they required hospitalization or surgery.

The results showed that those people who rated their health as poor were almost three times more likely to die during the seven years of the study than those who perceived their health to be excellent. Surprisingly, subjective self-reported health was more accurate in predicting who would die than the objective health measures from physicians. Those who were in objectively poor health by physician report survived at a higher rate as long as *they believed their own health to be good.*

Nearly 15 percent of the people rated their health as fair or poor, even though according to the objective health measures it was excellent or good. These "health pessimists" had a slightly greater risk of dying than the "health optimists" who viewed themselves as healthy in spite of negative reports from their doctors. The predictive power of self-rated health was the same whether one was male or female, older or younger, urban or rural, objectively sick or well. Only increasing age appeared to have a more powerful influence on death rates than self-rated health.

Another study of seven thousand adults in Alameda County in California confirmed the importance of the way a person views his health. Men with poor self-rated health were 2.3 times more likely to die than those who saw their health as excellent. For women the difference was five times greater. The importance of self-reported health remained even when health behaviors (smoking, drinking, and exercising), social ties (marriage and contacts with friends), and psychological state (happiness and depression) were accounted for.

If the association of self-rated health to risk of death is not entirely due to physical health status, health habits, or social connectedness, then what are the pathways by which it operates? It is possible that people have a very sensitive neural-sensing mechanism which detects subtle changes in health before symptoms appear and before a doctor can detect any dysfunctioning. Or a person's attitude about his own health may influence his future health—pessimistic attitudes are somehow translated into physiological dysfunctioning while optimism may even override underlying disease.

Positive attitudes seem to bolster the individual's ability to resist disease: Those with better self-reported health were less likely to die. Whatever the mechanism, the message is clear that how people view their own health significantly influences health outcomes. Of course there are limits to the effect of mental attitudes on physiological health; sometimes the biological disruption of advanced disease predominates.

Nevertheless, with all the emphasis on medical technology and diagnostic evaluation, let's not forget to inquire about what the most sophisticated diagnostic machine, the brain, has to say about health. Quickly assessing a person's overall perception of his health may tell us whether he is at greater risk. Who knows, perhaps by encouraging more positive self-perceptions we may be able to effect physiological processes and improve health outcomes.

Stressors are only one part of the equation for determining who maintains health and who gets ill. Resistance resources ranging from social support to hardiness, from coping strategies to belief in oneself, can have profound effects on whether one moves toward illness or health. But what are the common characteristics of these resistance resources which seem to promote good health?

Aaron Antonovsky, an Israeli medical sociologist, was first struck by the importance of resistance resources when he was conducting a study of how women from different ethnic backgrounds experienced and adapted to menopause. He identified a group of women who had been in the Nazi concentration camps during World War II. Not surprisingly, he found that the concentration camp survivors, as a group, were in poorer emotional and physical health than other women who had not been in the camps.

This is where such studies most often end, but Antonovsky looked more deeply. He was intrigued that some women survived the concentration camps and were healthy by all measures of physical, psychological, and social functioning. As he remarked, "Despite having lived through the most inconceivably inhuman experience, some women were reasonably healthy and happy, had raised families, worked, had friends, and were involved in community activities." How was this possible?

Antonovsky proposed that resistance resources which promote health, whether they be money, friends, education, or coping strategies, all worked to forge and reinforce a certain way of looking at the world, a way of perceiving the stimuli and demands which bombard the person. He originally defined this as a *sense of coherence*.

A sense of coherence is a global orientation that expresses the extent to which one has a pervasive, enduring though dynamic feeling of confidence that one's internal and external environments are predictable and that there is a high probability that things will work out as well as can reasonably be expected.

The sense of coherence includes three basic attributes: comprehensibility, manageability, and meaningfulness. *Comprehensibility* means that the demands made on the person seem ordered, consistent, structured, clear, and hence predictable, as opposed to random, chaotic, disordered, and unpredictable. *Manageability* refers to the extent to which people feel that they have resources at their disposal adequate to meet the demands made upon them. This does not mean that they have to control the resources—they could be controlled by friends, relatives, benevolent leaders, or God—but one way or the other, they will have access to adequate resources to help them cope. *Meaningfulness* refers to the feeling that the demands posed by living are viewed as worth investing in and worthy of commitment and engagement. The demands are meaningful in the sense that they are viewed as worthwhile challenges, not threats or unwelcome burdens.

A strong sense of coherence can function in many ways to strengthen health. The beliefs that life is meaningful, that one has the resources to cope with, and that life is ordered and predictable may allow one to engage in activities that are more health-promoting and avoid those that endanger health. This way of appraising the world may permit a person to see unavoidable stressors as challenges rather than threats and thereby short-circuit a stress reaction. Further, people with a stronger sense of coherence may be more likely to mobilize and effectively utilize resistance resources such as friends, material resources, and coping skills to deal with potentially stressful situations.

These psychological processes have their counterparts in brain function. Remember that the primary task of the brain and nervous system is to organize the world in order to increase the likelihood of survival. The brain selects only small bits of information from all the stimuli that reach us, organizes them into the most likely meaningful pattern, and remembers only a small organized sample of what has occurred. At each step the world becomes more organized and simplified in the mind. A network of schemata is developed to represent the chaotic and changing external world so that it becomes stable, simplified, and seemingly coherent in the mind. Instead of gray stone, thousands of reflecting bits of glass, scores of doors opening and closing, and several high ceilings, we perceive *one* building. The parts fit together. It makes sense.

We develop this stable organization (coherence), and it is basic to us in our connections to others. When this sense of coherence regarding a person's world is disrupted, he or she is more likely to become ill. If the world is disorganized, it is not clear what appropriate action to take in any situation, and it is not clear that we can control our lives to any extent. More importantly, it probably leads to conflict and confusion as the many different "small brains" within us vie for control. It can end in revolution outside or inside, in sudden changes in the world or sudden death.

There have always been, and will probably always be, two basic approaches to health: prevention and treatment. In ancient Greece they were symbolized by the two daughters of the healing god Asclepius. His one daughter, Panakeia, was knowledgeable in the use of medications to treat diseases. She is embodied today in the ongoing search for panaceas, drugs or treatments for all diseases. The other daughter, Hygea, was expert in teaching the ways of living in concert with nature in order to prevent disease.

This book has had a lot of emphasis on the search for ways to strengthen the resistance to disease and promote health. Although it focused on the role of the brain in health maintenance, its authors recognize that many other factors, from genes to germs, money to molecules, pollutants to politics, and diets to doctors, contribute to health. Further, brain states, mental attitudes, and emotional states, while partially controllable by the individual, are profoundly shaped by the physical and social worlds we live in.

At times we have been critical of an overdependence on a narrow mechanical view of medical care. We recognize that the healing capacities of the brain are not limitless. Wishes can make some things so, but not everything. Positive expectations may help relieve the pain of dental surgery but do little or nothing to reverse the biological disorder of advanced malignancy. The psychological determinants of health appear to have their maximum effect in maintaining health and preventing disease. In spite of biomedicine's best efforts to understand health and to support the brain in its healing function, there will always be breakdowns and the need for technical medical care.

The patient with cancer, heart disease, or any of scores of other disorders would be well advised not to skip medical care in favor of mental therapies. However, medical interventions can be applied in concert with the new understanding of the human brain as the primary health-maintenance organization. Attending to the psychological needs of the patient can complement the technical focus of modern biomedicine and may yield tremendous dividends in terms of comfort, decreased anxiety, and even recovery. Viewing the person in a broader social context is fully compatible and consistent with good medical practice. It is not either-or, body or mind. We are not built like that, and medical care should reflect our true unity.

An essential ingredient in promoting health seems to be the maintenance of stability inside one's body and a sense of stability about the external world. The human brain evolved to organize the world so that critical instabilities which represent threats to health and survival might be identified. The brain reduces the ever-changing, "blooming, buzzing confusion" of the real world to a stable, organized model. It does so by radically selecting sensory information, refining and processing it and, finally, organizing it into a workable set of routines which can encompass the world. Against this backdrop the brain then attempts to note changes or instabilities like an irregular beating of the heart or a bear approaching—irregularities which most likely signal danger.

Throughout the book we identified the many different factors which contribute to this vital sense of stability. One can even describe an idealized environment and life that might favor this sense of stability and health. The early childhood environment should foster strong bonding with the primary caregiver and other significant caregivers. These relationships should remain strong and supportive throughout life. The family should have strong routines which organize the days and years into predictable, persistent patterns.

One should live in a quiet, secure environment which changes slowly, if at all, and should have a strong sense of place or sense of being at home in familiar surroundings. The society should have strong, clear cultural beliefs and values with a strong social organization in which people know their place. A stable network of relatives, friends, and community members should be available to offer emotional support, advice, assistance, material resources, and opportunity for exchange of love and affection. When changes do occur, they should be gradual and incremental and should always be buffered by other sources of continuity and stability.

Boring, eh?

This fanciful portrait may show a life which supports mental stability and health, but it is more than a little out of touch with the realities of modern life faced by most of us. Avoiding change and social disruption is certainly one way to help stabilize the brain and insure health. Yet this approach yields a picture of health which seems to require that people lead quiet, rigid, lives, remain well integrated socially, and never rebel against the existing social order or produce any kind of innovation which upsets stability. It may be true that such a life *is* good for health in the sense of promoting a long, relatively disease-free life. Still, except for increasingly rare pastoral societies or in eras long gone, this approach to stability is not very possible.

People simply have other agendas and priorities than a long life. Consider the viewpoint expressed in the following quip from the newspaper:

> Statistically, single people earn less, go to jail twice as often, come down more frequently with ailments, kill themselves at a much greater rate, and certainly die at an earlier age. When a happily married man pointed that out, a confirmed bachelor drew the only conclusion obvious to him: If he wanted a long, lingering death he could get married.

Individual physical health is not necessarily the only or highest human value. In fact, many people are willing to sacrifice health in the pursuit of other goals. And there are many ways of maintaining stability which might not be in concert with other desired values. Totalitarian governments and cults might offer a strong, stable, organized social world supportive of health, but at some cost.

Another approach to stability is not to try to assume the world is static. Friends come and go, people move, people die, ideas change, people change. If one's entire sense of stability rests on such shifting sands, one is likely to be highly vulnerable. Human life has changed since the brain's priorities were set up. More people will be added to the earth in the next few years than lived at the time of Christ. We have space travel, computers, and more. The same brain processes which, after all, created this different world can certainly be used to comprehend it.

It is possible to find stability and learn to live in a rapidly changing world by regarding *change* as what is stable. When changes are immediately perceived as threats, this upsets the stability of the organism because the change cannot be comfortably incorporated into one's view of oneself or the world. However, changes understood as challenges, as opportunities for growth, can be incorporated into a stable, yet flexible, sense of the world. This requires an enormous cognitive and emotional flexibility. The ability to attach and strongly bond with others needs to be counterbalanced by the ability to detach and shift one's perspective.

If this approach is beginning to sound familiar, it is because it has been a part of traditional philosophies and religious teachings since earliest times. The medical systems of many ancient and traditional societies were carriers of this perennial philosophy.

People can learn to transcend the normal range of human reactions and knowledge. In many ways this achieves stability at a more organized level. Religious and spiritual figures describe a view of life as an organized process and our local hysteria, fads, and concerns as deviations and minor disruptions. Again, this is not such an esoteric perception as one might think, nor is it far away from much contemporary thought about health. Dr. Robert Eliot, who has worked with the heart attack–prone "hot reactors," advises just such a shift in perspective when he says that the heart patient (or the one who would rather not be a heart patient) has to learn: 1) Don't sweat the small stuff; and 2) It's all small stuff.

Relationships with people, pets, and plants; activities which draw us out of a narrow concern with ourselves into a larger involvement with life; and philosophies, cultural beliefs, and religions which enable us to see how our lives fit into a larger picture may protect our health. These pursuits involve a shift in

one's organization of the world, away from a focus on the scur-
ryings of daily events, and toward a more stable, complete view
of life on Earth, in which there will always be change, separation
and loss, and death of individuals, but life itself and our contribution to it will continue.

This viewpoint has usually been associated with many philo-
sophical and religious perspectives. It is put into action by encouraging service to others and a loss of self-centeredness. It is
common to almost all major religions. But perhaps it has less to
do with the ephemeral than scientists thought. It may be seen as
well-developed adaptations which lead to a stabler, healthier way
to view ourselves, our lives, and our place in society. That the
words *whole, heal,* and *holy* come from the same root is probably
not an accident. Seeing things whole makes them organized and
stable. Idries Shah, a man who is perhaps the most sophisticated
commentator on the relationship of the traditional psychologies
to modern life, recently observed:

> The human being is, almost by definition, one who doesn't know
> what is going to happen tomorrow—whether he is going to be run
> over by a streetcar in two minutes or drop dead in five.
> The human being does, in fact, live a transient life. But what he
> tries to do is to pretend that life is constant. What he can actually do
> is recognize that life is not constant—even solid objects are not solid
> and so on. He can be prepared for change so that change does not
> cause stress reactions, ulcers and worse.

It all works together: the countless adjustments of the heart;
the control of the immune system; the secretion of chemicals to
communicate within the brain and between the brain and the
organs; the stability of temperature, fluids, and food; the stability
of the person and the world outside; plans and performances; cell
to self to society. But we are just scratching the surface of a view
which can precisely encompass all these separate levels of reality.

We might, if we understood what brain mechanisms are for,
begin a new era for the management of individual and social
health, brain and health science. From an individual point of
view, we might be able to understand how our brain is a marvel-
ously flexible device and how it has enabled human beings and
our ancestors, through countless billions of operations, to create
the day-to-day world we live in. Understanding the brain may

help us see ways to change our idea of the world and, thereby, change our health.

Brain science is at the point, we believe, where medical science was before the emergence of the germ theory of disease. We have, for the first time, a way to think about the countless actions the brain takes: the billions of neural firings per second, the thousands of chemicals being secreted and sent all over the body, all the messages through the many branches of the nervous systems, immune systems, and circulatory systems of the body. They are health messages! The brain is there to keep us healthy.

Toward the end of his life, Albert Schweitzer was asked about his respect for traditional African medicine and so-called witch doctors. He responded, "The witch doctor succeeds for the same reason all the rest of us succeed. Each patient carries his own doctor inside him. They come to us not knowing that cure. We are at our best when we give the doctor who resides within each patient a chance to go to work."

For those who treat people as well as those being treated, the lesson is clear: The most important ally in the healing process is the patient, who is not merely a consumer of something dispensed to him as "health care" but is an organism developed over millennia and who possesses the most comprehensive healing instrument, the human brain.

NOTES

Preface

PAGE

11 In the early 1980s we developed through the Institute for the Study of Human Knowledge an ongoing series of symposia called *The Healing Brain*. These programs have been offered across the United States in cosponsorship with university extensions and medical school continuing education programs. Audiocassette tapes have been prepared on many of the topics and are available through ISHK Book Service, Box 1062, Cambridge, MA 02239.

Chapter 1: In Sickness and in Health

19 For a superb discussion of the determinants of health which contrasts the engineering model of modern medicine with a more ecological approach see J. Powles, On the limitations of modern medicine, *Science, Medicine and Man* 1 (1973):1–30. Abridged and reprinted in D. S. Sobel, ed., *Ways of Health: Holistic Approaches to Ancient and Contemporary Medicine* (New York: Harcourt Brace Jovanovich, 1979).

20 For a fascinating account of the history of infectious diseases and their impact on history see William H. McNeill, *Plagues and Peoples* (New York: Doubleday, 1976). The specific accounts and quotes are from Fernand Braudel's magnificent work, *Civilization and Capitalism in the Fifteenth–Eighteenth Centuries*, vol. 1, *The Structures of*

Everyday Life: The Limits of the Possible (New York: Harper & Row, 1984). Thomas McKeown offers the most thorough analysis of the reasons for the remarkable improvements in health in the past few centuries. He argues that the decline in infectious disease mortality for the most part occurred before the introduction of specific medical interventions and is better explained by improvements in nutrition, sanitation, and behavior. For example, see T. McKeown, *The Role of Medicine: Dream, Mirage or Nemesis?* (Princeton, NJ: Princeton University Press, 1979); and T. McKeown, Man's health: The past and the future, *Western Journal of Medicine* 132 (1980):49–57. J. B. McKinlay and S. M. McKinlay, The questionable contribution of medical measures to the decline of mortality in the United States in the twentieth century, *Milbank Memorial Fund Quarterly* 55 (1977):405–428. For a defense of the importance of biomedical research (not the practice of medicine), see S. Schneyer, J. S. Landeefeld, and F. H. Sandifer, Biomedical research and illness: 1900–1979, *Milbank Memorial Fund Quarterly* 59 (1981):44–59. For a defense of the important contribution of medical care to the improvement of health, see W. McDermott, Medicine: The public good and one's own, *Cornell University Medical College Alumni Quarterly* 40 (1977):15–24.

25 K. Steel, P. M. Gertman, and C. Crescenzi et al., Iatrogenic illness on a general medical service at a university hospital, *New England Journal of Medicine* 304 (1981):638–42. R. L. Kane, Iatrogenesis: Just what the doctor ordered, *Journal of Community Health* 5 (1980):149–158. A. B. Bergman and S. J. Stamm, The morbidity of cardiac "non-disease" in schoolchildren, *New England Journal of Medicine* 276 (1967):1008–13. G. Cayler et al., The effect of cardiac "non-disease" on intellectual and perceptual motor development, *British Heart Journal* 35 (1973):543.

25 The analysis of the comparative health of Utah and Nevada is from V. R. Fuchs, *Who Shall Live?* (New York: Basic Books, 1974).

26 The Alameda County Human Population Laboratory study on health habits is reported in N. B. Belloc and L. Breslow, Relationship of physical health status and health practices, *Preventive Medicine* 1 (1972):409–21; and N. B. Belloc, Relationship of health practices and mortality, *Preventive Medicine* 2 (1973):67–81.

27 For a critique of the reductionism of biomedicine and argument for a broader view of the determinants of health and disease, see G. L. Engel, The need for a new medical model: A challenge for biomedicine, *Science* 196 (1977):129–36. G. L. Engel, The clinical application of the biopsychosocial model, *American Journal of Psychiatry* 137

(1980):535–44. R. Dubos, *Man Adapting* (New Haven: Yale University Press, 1965). R. Dubos, *Mirage of Health* (New York: Doubleday & Co., 1959).

28 R. Dubos, *Louis Pasteur: Free Lance of Science* (New York: C. H. Scribner's Sons, 1976). R. Dubos, Bolstering the body against disease, *Human Nature* (August 1978):68–72.

29 T. Ishigami, The influence of psychic acts on the progress of pulmonary tuberculosis, *American Review of Tuberculosis* 2 (1919):470–84. T. H. Holmes, N. G. Hawkins, C. E. Bowerman, E. R. Clarke, and J. R. Joffe, Psychosocial and psychophysiologic studies of tuberculosis, *Psychosomatic Medicine* 19 (1957):134–43. J. B. Jemmott and S. E. Locke, Psychosocial factors, immunologic mediation and human susceptibility to infectious diseases: How much do we know? *Psychological Bulletin* 95 (1984):78–108.

31 For a discussion of the limits of risk factors in predicting who will develop heart disease, see S. L. Syme, Social support and risk reduction, *Mobius* 4 (1984):44–54. Pooling Project Research Group, Relationship of blood pressure, serum cholesterol, smoking habit, relative weight, and ECG abnormalities to incidence of major coronary events: Final report on the Pooling Project, *Journal of Chronic Disease* 31 (1978):201–306.

Chapter 2: Bodyguards

36 The most influential work on homeostasis is W. Cannon, *Bodily Changes in Pain, Hunger, Fear and Rage: An Account of Recent Researches into the Function of Emotional Excitement*, 2nd ed. (New York: Appleton-Century-Crofts, 1929). A general review of brain regulation of physiological processes can be found in C. Cotman and J. McGaugh, *Behavioral Neuroscience* (New York: Academic Press, 1980).

36 See R. Ornstein, R. Thompson, and D. Macaulay, *The Amazing Brain* (Boston: Houghton Mifflin Co., 1984) for a full treatment of how the brain evolved.

38 For a discussion of how the senses function to select information coming in, see R. Ornstein, *The Psychology of Consciousness* (New York: Viking-Penguin, 1986); and E. Galanter, Contemporary psychophysics, in *New Directions in Psychology* ed. R. Brown, E. Galanter, E. Hess, and G. Mandler (New York: Holt, Rinehart & Winston, 1982) pp. 85–157.

42 For a more detailed description of the priority system see R. Ornstein, *Multimind* (Boston: Houghton Mifflin Co., 1986).

42 A. Maslow, *Motivation and Personality* (New York: Harper & Row, 1970).

43 A. Borquist, Crying, *American Journal of Psychology* 17 (1906):149–205.

44 W. H. Frey II, D. DeSota-Johnson, C. Hoffman, and J. T. McCall, Effect of stimulus on the chemical composition of human tears, *American Journal of Ophthalmology* 92:4 (1981):559–67.

44 C. Dinarello and S. Wolfe, Fever, *Human Nature* 2:2 (1979):66–74.

49 B. K. Anand and J. R. Brobeck, Hypothalamic control of food intake in rats and cats, *Yale Journal of Biology and Medicine* 24 (1951):123–140.

49 S. Grossman, The biology of motivation, *Annual Review of Psychology* 30 (1979):209–42. A. W. Hetherington and S. W. Ranson, The spontaneous activity and food intake of rats with hypothalamic lesions, *American Journal of Physiology* 136 (1942):609–17.

50 For a clear treatment of the set point idea see William Bennett and J. Gurin, *Dieter's Dilemma: Eating Less and Weighing More* (New York: Basic Books, 1982); and a series of audiocassette tapes by William Bennett, *Set Point Regulation of Body Weight*, ISHK Tapes, Box 1062, Cambridge, MA 02239.

52 R. Andres, D. Elahi, J. D. Tobin, D. C. Muller, and L. Brant, Impact of age on weight goals, *Annals of Internal Medicine* 103:6, part 2 (1985):1030–33.

Chapter 3: The Self-ish Brain

56 For a discussion of how sensory information is limited, selected, and then constructed into a model of reality and how the senses and the brain are built to respond to changes see R. Ornstein, *The Psychology of Consciousness*.

57 For a full description of the talents of the "small minds" that make up the brain and how the mind "wheels," see R. Ornstein, *Multimind* (Boston: Houghton Mifflin Co., 1986).

59 The most relevant work on the frontal lobes is by W. J. H. Nauta, The problem of the frontal lobe: A reinterpretation, *Journal of Psychiatric Research* 8 (1971):167–87. W. J. H. Nauta, Neural associations of the frontal cortex, *Acta Neurobiologiae Experimentalis* 32 (1972):125–140. W. J. H. Nauta, Connections of the frontal lobe with the limbic system, in *Surgical approaches in psychiatry* ed. L. V. Laitinen and R. E. Livingston (Baltimore: University Park Press, 1973).

60 For a full description of the function of the two cerebral hemispheres see R. Ornstein, *The Psychology of Consciousness;* and D. Galin and R. Ornstein, Lateral specialization of cognitive mode: An EEG study, *Psychophysiology* 9 (1972):412–18. D. Galin, R. E. Ornstein, J. Herron, and J. Johnstone, Sex and handedness differences in EEG measures of hemispheric specialization, *Brain and Language,* 16:1 (1982):19–55.

61 See the work out of Richard Davidson's laboratory for the most interesting research. An early study is described in R. Davidson, Hemispheric asymmetry and emotion, in *Approaches to Emotion* ed. K. Scherer and P. Ekman (Hillsdale, NJ: Lawrence Erlbaum, 1984).

63 The laboratory of Paul Ekman has begun to revolutionize the study of emotion. See P. Ekman, Expression and the nature of emotion, in *Approaches to Emotion* ed. K. Scherer and P. Ekman (Hillsdale, NJ: Lawrence Erlbaum, 1984).

63 The seminal book on emotions was written more than one hundred years ago by Charles Darwin. C. Darwin, *The Expression of the Emotions in Man and Animals* (Chicago: University of Chicago Press, 1965).

67 C. Osgood et al., *The Measurement of Meaning* (Urbana: University of Illinois Press, 1971).

General note to this chapter: The emergence of "self" is difficult to measure, but some evidence is found in G. G. Gallup, Self-recognition in primates: A comparative approach to the bi-directional properties of consciousness, *American Psychologist* 32 (1977):329–38. G. G. Gallup, Self-awareness in primates, *American Scientist* 67 (1979):417–21.

Chapter 4: The Powerful Placebo

74 Jerome Frank offers an excellent analysis of the powerful psychological factors at work in religious healing shrines. See J. Frank, *Persuasion and Healing* (Baltimore: Johns Hopkins Press, 1973).

75 For another version of this tongue-in-cheek description of The Johns Hopkins School of Medicine and Hospitals see Frank's commencement address to the medical students published in Jerome Frank, The faith that heals, *The Johns Hopkins Medical Journal* 137 (1975):127–31.

76 The best current reference on placebos is L. White, B. Tursky, and G. E. Schwartz, eds., *Placebo: Theory, Research and Mechanisms* (New York: The Guilford Press, 1985). This book contains twenty-five papers and discussions of the many facets of the placebo effect.

77 Arthur Shapiro, a pioneer in the current investigation of the placebo effect, noted that until recent times most of the history of medicine can be regarded as the history of the placebo effect. See A. K. Shapiro, A contribution to the history of the placebo effect, *Behavioral Science* 5 (1960):109–35; and A. K. Shapiro, Factors contributing to the placebo effect, *American Journal of Psychotherapy* 73 (1964):73–88.

77 The "natural history"—what will happen if no treatment or intervention is applied—is extremely important to the evaluation of the efficacy of any treatment, including placebos. Often experiments and clinical trials are performed using placebos alone as the control, which leaves open the question of what would happen if no treatment, including placebos, were applied. See H. L. Fields and J. D. Levine, Biology of placebo analgesia, *American Journal of Medicine* 70 (1981):745–46.

79 H. K. Beecher, The powerful placebo, *Journal of the American Medical Association* 159 (1955):1602–6. In considering Beecher's finding that on average a third of patients will respond to a placebo, it must be noted that this is an average figure. Depending on the patients, disease, and treatment conditions the actual response may vary from 0 to almost 100 percent. See A. K. Shapiro and L. A. Morris, The placebo effect in medical and psychological therapies, in *The Handbook of Psychotherapy and Behavior Change*, 2d ed., ed. S. L. Garfield and A. E. Bergin (New York: John Wiley, 1978).

79 For a good brief review of the placebo effect in various diseases see H. Benson and M. D. Epstein, The placebo effect: A neglected asset in the care of patients, *Journal of the American Medical Association* 232 (1975):1225–26.

79 Stewart Wolf conducted a series of experiments demonstrating that many "drug effects" are not due to pharmacological action but to psychological factors. "Placebo effects which modify the pharmacological action of drugs or endow inert agents with potency are not imaginary, but may be associated with measurable changes at the end organs. These effects are at times more potent than the pharmacological action customarily attributed to the agent." See S. Wolf, Effects of suggestion and conditioning on the action of chemical agents in human subjects: The pharmacology of placebos, *Journal of Clinical Investigation* 29 (1950):100–109.

79 For a review of placebo-induced side effects, sometimes referred to as *nocebo effects*, see A. K. Shapiro and L. A. Morris, The placebo effect in medical and psychological therapies, in *The Handbook of*

Psychotherapy and Behavior Change, 2d ed., ed. S. L. Garfield and A. E. Bergin (New York: John Wiley, 1978).

80 For a review of the placebo effect in surgery see H. K. Beecher, Surgery as placebo: A quantitative study of bias, *Journal of the American Medical Association* 176 (1961):1102–07; and H. Benson and D. P. McCallie, Angina pectoris and the placebo effect, *New England Journal of Medicine* 300 (1979):1424–29.

81 For a discussion of the nonspecific psychological effects of coronary bypass surgery see J. Frank, The faith that heals, *The Johns Hopkins Medical Journal* 137 (1975): 127–31.

82 Many theories have been proposed to explain whether or not a placebo will work and who will respond. For instance, there is a considerable amount of evidence that suggests that the "placebo reactor" is highly suggestible, hysterical, neurotic, dependent, weak-willed, and introverted. However, there is an equally impressive number of studies that indicate quite contradictory findings from these. At present, there is no reliable description of the personality of a placebo responder. In fact, we find that a person who responds to a placebo in one situation may fail to respond in another. For a discussion of some of the explanations of placebo response see Shapiro and Morris, The placebo effect in medical and psychological therapies; and White, Tursky, and Schwartz, *Placebo: Theory, Research and Mechanisms*.

82 H. Rheder, Wunderheilungen, ein experiment, *Hippokrates* 26 (1955):577–80. Described in J. Frank, Mind-body relationships in illness and healing, *Journal of the International Academy of Preventive Medicine* 2 (1975):46–59.

82 H. K. Beecher, Relationship of significance of wound to pain experienced, *Journal of the American Medical Association* 161 (1956): 1609–13.

83 S. L. Gryll and M. Katahn, Situational factors contributing to the placebo effect, *Psychopharmacology* 57 (1978):253–61.

84 L. D. Egbert, Postscript, *Advances* 2 (1985):56–9.

84 N. Fiore, Fighting cancer: One patient's perspective, *New England Journal of Medicine* 300 (1979):284–89.

85 W. S. Agras, M. Horne, and C. B. Taylor, Expectation and the blood-pressure-lowering effect of relaxation, *Psychosomatic Medicine* 44 (1982):389–95.

86 For a discussion of the confusing literature on the effect of physical characteristics of placebos (size, color, taste, route of administration), see L. W. Buckalew and S. Ross, Relationship of
perceptual characteristics to efficacy of placebos, *Psychological Reports* 49 (1981):955–61.

86 A. Branthwaite and P. Cooper, Analgesic effect of branding in
treatment of headaches, *British Medical Journal* 282 (1981):1576–78.

87 There are serious ethical barriers to the use of placebos centering
on the deception of the patient by the physician, even if the deception is intended to aid the patient. (See, for example, S. Bok, The
ethics of giving placebos, *Scientific American* 231 (1974):17–23.) The
widespread use of placebos might also relieve symptoms caused by
serious disease and thus delay appropriate diagnostic studies and
treatment. Contrary to what many physicians believe, the response
of a patient to a placebo does not support the view that the patient's
symptoms were due to psychogenic rather than organic causes (see
J. S. Goodwin, J. M. Goodwin, and A. V. Vogel, Knowledge and
use of placebos by house officers and nurses, *Annals of Internal
Medicine* 91 (1979):106–10).

87 Norman Cousins, in his book *Anatomy of an Illness as Perceived by the
Patient* (New York: W. W. Norton, 1980), offers an account of his
own experience with a crippling arthritic condition. He attributes
part of his remarkable recovery to his ability to mobilize positive
emotions and discusses the placebo effect as testimony to the
power of mental states in healing.

Chapter 5: The Pharmacy Within

89 For a fuller discussion of the chemical nature of the brain see Ornstein, Thompson, and Macauley, *The Amazing Brain*.

91 A. Goldstein, Thrills in response to music and other stimuli, *Physiological Psychology* 8 (1980):126–29.

93 Endorphins do not mediate all the intrinsic pain relief systems. For
example, naloxone has not been shown to block hypnotic analgesia. Also other neurotransmitters, such as the catecholamines, are
thought to be involved in some nonopioid pain relief pathways.
See J. C. Liebeskind et al., Our natural capacities for pain suppression, *Advances* 1 (1983):8–11.

96 J. D. Levine, N. C. Gordon, and H. L. Fields, The mechanism of
placebo analgesia, *Lancet* 2 (1978):654–57; J. D. Levine, N. C. Gordon, J. C. Bornstein, and H. L. Fields, Role of pain in placebo
analgesia, *Proceedings of the National Academy of Sciences* 76

(1979):3528–31; and J. D. Levine, N. C. Gordon, R. T. Jones, and H. L. Fields, The narcotic antagonist naloxone enhances clinical pain, *Nature* 272 (1978):826.

97 J. D. Levine and N. C. Gordon, Influence of the method of drug administration on analgesic response, *Nature* 312 (1984):755–56.

97 In addition to pain suppression, endorphins appear to effect mood, appetite, and immunity. Endorphins are also produced in tissues other than brain such as those in the gut.

Chapter 6: Great Expectations

99 For an account of Hilgard's interesting work with hypnosis and consciousness see E. R. Hilgard, *Divided Consciousness: Multiple Controls in Human Thought and Action* (New York: Wiley-Interscience, 1977); and E. R. Hilgard, Hypnosis and consciousness, *Human Nature* 1:1 (1978):42–51.

99 For a superb review of how bodily function can be altered by suggestion see T. X. Barber, Changing "unchangeable" bodily processes by (hypnotic) suggestions: A new look at hypnosis, cognitions, imagining, and the mind-body problem, *Advances* 1 (1984):7–36.

100 The case of Holly is presented in O. S. Surman, S. K. Gottlieb, and T. P. Hackett, Hypnotic treatment of a child with warts, *American Journal of Clinical Hypnosis* 15 (1972):12–14. Another more recent case history of successful wart regression is presented in B. A. Morris, Hypnotherapy of warts using the Simonton visualization technique: A case report, *American Journal of Clinical Hypnosis* 27 (1983):237–40. The ten-year-old patient was hypnotized and given the suggestion that the "food supply to the warts" was being cut off and that she should imagine that her own white blood cells were attacking and destroying them. The patient reported having a number of spontaneous daydreams in which she saw "little guys in white coats with black buckles and big sticks, marching and attacking the warts." Within three months all fifty of the warts on her hands had regressed. The warts had been present for three years prior to hypnotherapy and had survived previous treatment of liquid nitrogen, curettage, and electrodessication.

101 Bruno Block, described in Barber, Changing "unchangeable" bodily processes by (hypnotic) suggestions, *Advances* 1 (1984): 7–36.

101 A. H. C. Sinclair-Gieben and D. Chalmers, Evaluation of treatment of warts by hypnosis, *Lancet* 2 (1959):480–82.

101 For details on the study at Massachusetts General Hospital, see O. S. Surman, S. K. Gottlieb, T. P. Hackett, and E. L. Silverberg, Hypnosis in the treatment of warts, *Archives of General Psychiatry* 28 (1973):439–41.

102 Lewis Thomas offers his plea for a serious study of warts, "the turreted mounds of dense impenetrable horn," which in spite of their look of toughness and permanence, can inexplicably and abruptly vanish due to "something like thinking." "Just think of what we would know if we had anything like a clear understanding of what goes on when a wart is hypnotized away. . . . We would be finding out about a kind of superintelligence that exists in each of us, infinitely smarter and possessed of technical know-how far beyond our present understanding. It would be worth a War on Warts, a Conquest of Warts, a National Institute of Warts and All." See Lewis Thomas: *The Medusa and the Snail* (New York: Viking, 1979).

102 R. D. Willard, Breast enlargement through visual imagery and hypnosis, *American Journal of Clinical Hypnosis* 19 (1977):195–200.

103 Y. Ikemi and S. Nakagawa, A psychosomatic study of contagious dermatitis, *Kyushu Journal of Medical Science* 13 (1962):335–50.

Chapter 7: Small Worlds, Small Brains

106 For a thorough account of how the sensory system reduces incoming input and how the brain constructs a model of reality see Ornstein, *The Psychology of Consciousness;* and J. E. Hochberg, *Perception,* 2d ed. (Englewood Cliffs, NJ: Prentice-Hall, 1978).

109 S. Schachter and J. Singer, Cognitive, social, and physiological determinants of emotional state, *Psychological Review* 69 (1962):379–99.

110 J. C. Speisman, R. S. Lazarus, L. Davidson, and A. M. Mordkoff, Experimental analysis of a film used as a threatening stimulus, *Journal of Consulting Psychology* 28:1 (1964):23–33.

112 For further discussion and examples of the importance of the symbolic reality of medicine and explanatory models see Sobel, *Ways of Health;* and A. Kleinman, *Patients and Healers in the Context of Culture* (Berkeley: University of California Press, 1980).

Chapter 8: People Need People

119 For an excellent recent review of the evidence linking social support and health, see S. Cohen and S. L. Syme, eds., *Social Support and Health* (New York: Academic Press, 1985). Also see W. E. Broadhead, B. H. Kaplan, S. A. James, E. H. Wagner, V. J. Schoenbach,

R. Grimson, S. Heyden, G. Tibblin, and S. H. Gehlbach, The epidemiological evidence for a relationship between social support and health, *American Journal of Epidemiology* 117 (1983):521–37. L. F. Berkman, Assessing the physical health effects of social networks and social support, *Annual Review of Public Health* 5 (1984):413–32.

120 E. Durkeim, *Suicide* (New York: Free Press, 1951).

121 W. B. Neser, H. A. Tyroler, and J. C. Cassel, Social disorganization and stroke mortality in the black population of North Carolina, *American Journal of Epidemiology* 93 (1971):166–75; and S. James and D. G. Kleinbaum, Socioecologic stress and hypertension: Related mortality rates in North Carolina, *American Journal of Public Health* 66 (1976):354–58.

122 M. H. Brenner, Importance of the economy to the nation's health. In *The Relevance of Social Science for Medicine*, ed. L. Eisenberg and A. Kleinman (Dordrecht, Holland: D. Reidel Pub. Co., 1980).

122 L. Berkman and S. L. Syme, Social networks, host resistance, and mortality: A nine-year follow-up study of Alameda County residents, *American Journal of Epidemiology* 109 (1979):186–204.

123 J. S. House, C. Robbins, and H. L. Metzner, The association of social relationships and activities with mortality, *American Journal of Epidemiology* 116 (1982):123–40.

124 J. C. Cassel, The contribution of the social environment to host resistance, *American Journal of Epidemiology* 104 (1976):107–23. S. L. Syme and L. F. Berkman, Social class, susceptibility and sickness, *American Journal of Epidemiology* 104 (1976):1–8. S. L. Syme, Sociocultural factors and disease etiology, in *Handbook of Behavioral Medicine*, ed. W. Doyle Gentry (New York: The Guilford Press, 1984).

125 M. G. Marmot and S. L. Syme, Acculturation and coronary heart disease in Japanese-Americans, *American Journal of Epidemiology* 104 (1976):225–47. M. G. Marmot, S. L. Syme, A. Kagan, H. Kato, J. B. Cohen and J. Belsky, Epidemiological studies of coronary heart disease and stroke in Japanese men living in Japan, Hawaii, and California: Prevalence of coronary and hypertensive heart disease and associated risk factors, *American Journal of Epidemiology* 102 (1975):514–25.

125 J. Brown, et al., Nutritional and Epidemiological factors related to heart disease, *World Review of Nutrition and Dietetics*, 12 (New York: Karger, 1970), pp. 1–42.

126 A discussion of the immigrant question is also found in J. Lynch, *The Broken Heart* (New York: Basic Books, 1977).

126 S. Gore, The effect of social support in moderating the health consequences of unemployment, *Journal of Health and Social Behavior* 19 (1978):157–65.

126 K. B. Nuckolls, J. C. Cassel, and B. H. Kaplan, Psychosocial assets, life crisis, and the prognosis of pregnancy, *American Journal of Epidemiology* 95 (1972):431–41.

127 G. W. Brown and T. Harris, *Social Origins of Depression* (New York: Free Press, 1978).

127 Teresa Seeman, Social support and angiography, doctoral thesis, University of California, Berkeley, 1985.

128 A. Beck and A. Katcher, *Between Pets and People: The Importance of Animal Companionship* (New York: G. P. Putnam, 1983). A. Katcher and A. Beck, eds., *New Perspectives on Our Lives with Companion Animals* (Philadelphia: University of Pennsylvania Press, 1983). F. T. FitzGerald, The therapeutic value of pets, *Western Journal of Medicine* 144 (1986):103–5. E. Friedmann, A. Katcher, J. J. Lynch, and S. A. Thomas, Animal companions and one-year survival of patients after discharge from a coronary care unit, *Public Health Reports* 95 (1980):307–12.

Chapter 9: From the Individual to the Social Body

132 Perhaps the most readable account of the discovery of our earliest ancestors is Don Johansen's book on Lucy. It contains also a stimulating discussion of adaptive virtues of bipedalism by Owen Lovejoy. D. Johansen and M. Edey, *Lucy: The Beginnings of Human Kind* (New York: Simon & Schuster, 1981).

132 For a popular account of the effect of brain and pelvis size on growth, see Roger Lewin and Richard Leakey's interesting book, *Origins* (New York: E. P. Dutton, 1977). See also J. B. S. Haldane, *The Causes of Evolution* (London: Longmans, Green, 1932) for a discussion of many of the major issues in biological evolution and for arresting quips.

133 Perhaps the most interesting discussion of the role that human fathers take is found in R. D. Alexander, J. L. Hoogland, R. D. Howard, K. M. Noonan, and P. W. Sherman, in *Evolutionary Biology and Human Social Behavior: An Anthropological Perspective*, ed. N. A. Chagnons and W. G. Irons (North Scituate, MA: Duxbury Press, 1979).

134 See, for instance, J. Bowlby, *Attachment and Loss*, vols. 1–3 (New York: Basic Books, 1969). Mary Ainsworth has developed a situa-

tion in which attachment can be studied. See M. D. S. Ainsworth, *Infancy in Uganda* (Baltimore: Johns Hopkins University Press, 1967). M. D. S. Ainsworth, and S. M. Bell, Attachment, exploration and separation: Illustrated by the behavior of one-year-olds in a strange situation, *Child Development* 41 (1970). M. D. S. Ainsworth, M. Blehar, E. Waters, and S. Wall, *Patterns of Attachment: A Psychological Study of the Strange Situation* (Hillsdale, NJ: Lawrence Erlbaum, 1978). M. D. S. Ainsworth and B. A. Wittig, Attachment and exploratory behavior of one-year-olds in a strange situation, in *Determinants of Infant Behavior*, vol. 4, ed. B. M. Foxx (London: Methuen, 1965).

Chapter 10: Mind-Made Immunity

139 R. W. Bartrop, L. Lazarus, E. Luckhurst, L. G. Kiloh, and R. Penny, Depressed lymphocyte function after bereavement, *Lancet* 1 (1977):834–39. Also see S. J. Schliefer, S. E. Keller, M. Camerino, J. C. Thornton, and M. Stein, Suppression of lymphocyte stimulation following bereavement, *Journal of the American Medical Association* 250 (1983):374–77.

140 For the lay reader the best current summary of the emerging field of psychoneuroimmunology is S. Locke and D. Colligan, *The Healer Within* (New York: E. P. Dutton, 1986). For a more technical discussion see R. Ader, ed., *Psychoneuroimmunology* (New York: Academic Press, 1981).

141 Some early reports linking the brain and immune function can be found in H. O. Besedovsky, A. Del Rey, E. Sorkin, M. DaPrada, and H. H. Keller, Immunoregulation mediated by the sympathetic nervous system, *Cell Immunology* 48 (1979):346. S. Black, J. H. Humphrey, and J. S. F. Niven, Inhibition of Mantoux reaction by direct suggestion under hypnosis, *British Medical Journal* 1 (1963):1649–52. G. F. Solomon and R. H. Moos, Emotions, immunity and disease: A speculative theoretical integration, *Archives of General Psychiatry* 11 (1964):657–74.

142 The first report of Ader's work is found in R. Ader and H. Cohen, Behaviorally conditioned immunosuppression, *Psychosomatic Medicine* 37 (1975):333–40. For a recent review including twenty-four peer commentaries and responses see R. Ader and N. Cohen, CNS-immune system interactions: Conditioning phenomena, *Brain and Behavioral Sciences* 8 (1985):379–426. Further reports are found in R. Ader and N. Cohen, Conditioned immunopharmacologic responses, in *Psychoneuroimmunology*, ed. R. Ader; R. Ader and N. Cohen, Behaviorally conditioned immunosuppression and mu-

rine systemic lupus erythematosus, *Science* 215 (1982):1534–36; R. Ader and N. Cohen, Behavior and the immune system, in *Handbook of Behavioral Medicine,* ed. D. Gentry; and D. Bovbjerg and R. Ader, Acquisition and extinction of conditioned suppression of a graft-vs.-host response in the rat, *Psychosomatic Medicine* 45 (1983):369 (abstract).

142 R. M. Gorczynski, S. Macrae, and M. Kennedy, Conditioned immune response associated with allogeneic skin grafts in mice, *Journal of Immunology* 129 (1982):704–9.

144 For a critical discussion of the links between measurements of immune function and the nervous system see T. Melnechuk, Why has psychoneuroimmunology been controversial? *Advances* 2 (1985): 22–38.

147 The case is drawn from D. L. Larson, *Systemic lupus erythematosus* (Boston: Little Brown & Co., 1961).

148 G. F. Solomon and R. H. Moos, The relationship of personality to the presence of rheumatoid factor in asymptomatic relatives of patients with rheumatoid arthritis, *Psychosomatic Medicine* 27 (1965):350–60.

148 For a review of the numerous connections between the nervous and immune systems see several of the chapters in R. Ader, *Psychoneuroimmunology* and G. F. Solomon, The emerging field of psychoneuroimmunology, *Advances* 2 (1985):6–19.

149 N. Geschwind and A. Galaburda, eds., *Biological Foundations of Cerebral Dominance* (Cambridge: Harvard University Press, 1984).

149 G. Renoux, K. Biziere, M. Renoux, and J. M. Guillamin, The production of T-cell-inducing factors in mice is controlled by the brain neocortex, *Scandinavian Journal of Immunology* 17 (1983):45–50.

150 E. A. Korneva and L. M. Khai, Effects of destruction of hypothalamic areas on immunogenesis, *Fiziol ZL SSSR* 49 (1963):42–46. E. A. Korneva, The effects of stimulating different mesencephalic structures on protective immune response pattern, *Fiziol ZL SSSR* 53 (1967):42–45. For a review see M. D. Stein, S. J. Schleifler, and S. E. Keller, Hypothalamic influences on immune responses, in *Psychoneuroimmunology,* ed. R. Ader.

150 H. O. Besedeovsky, E. Sorkin, D. Felix, and H. Haas, Hypothalamic changes during the immune response, *European Journal of Immunology* 7 (1977):325–28. Besedovsky, del Rey, et al., Immunoregulation mediated by the sympathetic nervous system. H. O.

Besedovsky, A. Del Ray, and E. Sorkin, What do the immune system and the brain know about each other? *Immunology Today* 4 (1983):342–46.

151 Y. Shavit, J. W. Lewis, G. W. Terman, R. P. Gale, and J. C. Liebeskind, Endogenous opioids may mediate the effects of stress on tumor growth and immune function, *Proceedings of the Western Pharmacological Society* 26 (1983):53–56.

151 V. Riley, M. A. Fitzmaurice, and D. H. Spackman, Psychoneuroimmunologic factors in neoplasia: Studies in animals, in *Psychoneuroimmunology*, ed. R. Ader.

152 M. L. Laudenslager, S. M. Ryan, R. C. Drugan, R. L. Hyson, and S. F. Maier, Coping and immunosuppression: Inescapable but not escapable shock suppresses lymphocyte proliferation, *Science* 221 (1983):568–70. Their review article is S. F. Maier and M. Laudenslager, Stress and health: Exploring the links, *Psychology Today* (August 1985):44–49.

152 J. D. Palmbad, Stress and immunologic competence: Studies in man, in *Psychoneuroimmunology*, ed. R. Ader.

153 S. V. Kasl, A. S. Evans, and J. C. Neiderman, Psychosocial risk factors in the development of infectious mononucleosis, *Psychosomatic Medicine* 41 (1979):445–66. For a review see J. B. Jemmott and S. E. Locke, Psychosocial factors, immunologic mediation and human susceptibility to infection: How much do we know? *Psychological Bulletin* 95 (1984):78–108.

153 D. D. Schmidt, S. Zyzanski, J. Ellner, M. L. Kumar, and J. Arno, Stress as a precipitating factor in subjects with recurrent herpes labialis, *Journal of Family Practice* 20 (1985):359–66.

154 J. K. Kiecolt-Glaser, W. Garner, C. Speicher, G. M. Penn, J. Holliday, and R. Glaser, Psychosocial modifiers of immunocompetence in medical students, *Psychosomatic Medicine* 46 (1984):7–14.

154 S. E. Locke, L. Kraus, J. Leserman, M. W. Hurst, J. S. Heisel, and R. M. Williams, Life change stress, psychiatric symptoms, and natural killer cell activity, *Psychosomatic Medicine* 46:5 (1984):441–53.

154 H. Hall, S. Longo, and R. Dixon, Hypnosis and the immune system: The effect of hypnosis on T and B cell function, presented to the Society for Clinical and Experimental Hypnosis, 33d Annual Workshops and Scientific Meeting, Portland, OR. Also see H. Hall, Hypnosis and the immune system: A review with implications for

cancer and the psychology of healing, *American Journal of Clinical Hypnosis* 25 (1983):92–103.

155 J. K. Kiecolt-Glaser, R. Glaser, et al., Psychosocial enhancement of immunocompetence in a geriatric population, *Health Psychology* 4 (1985):25–41.

155 David McClelland and his coworkers have been among the most interesting groups researching psychological and immune effects. For a wide-ranging and stimulating interview with McClelland see J. Z. Borysenko, Healing motives: An interview with David McClelland, *Advances* 2 (1985):29–41. The quote on pages 159–60 is from this interview. Related studies include D. C. McClelland, G. Ross, and V. Patel, The effect of an academic examination on salivary norepinephrine and immunoglobulin levels, *Journal of Human Stress*, 11 (1985):52–59. D. C. McClelland, E. Floor, R. J. Davidson, and C. Saron, Stressed power motivation, sympathetic activation, immune function, and illness, *Journal of Human Stress* 6 (1980): 11–19. D. C. McClelland and J. B. Jemmott, Power motivation, stress and physical illness, *Journal of Human Stress* 6 (1980):6–15. J. B. Jemmott, J. Z. Borysenko, M. Borysenko, D. C. McClelland, R. Chapman, D. Meyer, and H. Benson, Academic stress, power motivation, and decrease in secretion rate of salivary secretory immunoglobulin A, *Lancet* (1983):1400–1402. D. C. McClelland, and C. Kirshnit, The effect of motivational arousal through films on salivary immune function, unpublished manuscript.

155 K. M. Dillon, B. Minchoff, and K. H. Baker, Positive emotional states and enhancement of the immune system, *International Journal of Psychiatry in Medicine* 15 (1985–86):13–17.

156 C. L. Coe, L. T. Rosenberg, and S. Levine, Effect of maternal separation on humoral immunity in infant primates, in Proceedings of the First International Workshop on Neuroimmunomodulation, Bethesda, MD, November 27–30, 1984, ed. N. H. Spector, See also M. Reite and T. Fields, eds., *The Psychobiology of Attachment and Separation* (New York: Academic Press, 1985).

157 L. Derogatis, M. Abeloff, and N. Melisaratos, Psychological coping mechanisms and survival time in metastatic breast cancer, *Journal of the American Medical Association* 242 (1979):1504–8.

157 The Norman Cousins description is from his introduction to Locke and Colligan, *The Healer Within.*

157 S. Greer and T. Morris, Psychological attributes of women who develop breast cancer, *Psychosomatic Research* 19 (1975):147–53.

H. S. Greer, T. Morris, and K. W. Pettingale, Psychological response to breast cancer: Effect on outcome, *Lancet* 2 (1979):785–87. For a discussion of emotions and cancer see also S. M. Levy, Emotions and the progression of cancer: A review, *Advances* 1 (1984): 10–15.

158 B. R. Cassileth, E. J. Lusk, D. S. Miller, L. L. Brown, and C. Miller, Psychosocial correlates of survival in advanced malignant disease? *New England Journal of Medicine* 312 (1985):1551–55. See also the letters to the editor in response, *New England Journal of Medicine* 313 (1986):1354–59.

Chapter 11: Pressure: Social and Blood

162 T. B. Graboys, Celtic fever: Playoff-induced ventricular arrythmia, *New England Journal of Medicine* 305 (1981):467–8.

163 The quote and material that follows is from James Lynch, *The Language of the Heart* (New York: Basic Books, 1985).

165 Some of the evidence on blood pressure comes from S. A. Thomas et al., Patients' cardiac responses to nursing interviews in a CCU, *Dimensions of Critical Care Nursing* 1:4 (July–August 1982):198–205. R. Coleman, M. Greenblatt, and H. Solomon, Physiological evidence of rapport during psychotherapeutic interviews, *Diseases of the Nervous System* 17 (1956):71–78. S. Wolf, Cardiovascular reactions to symbolic stimuli, *Circulation* 18 (1958):287–92. H. Weiner, *The Psychobiology of Hypertension* (New York: Elsevier, 1979). S. A. Thomas et al., Blood pressure and heart rate changes in children when they read aloud in school, *Public Health Reports* 99:1 (1984): 77–84.

166 G. Mancia, G. Grassi, G. Pomidossi, et al., Effects of blood pressure measurement by the doctor on patient's blood pressure and heart rate, *Lancet* (September 24, 1983):695–98.

166 E. Lynch et al., Blood pressure and heart rate increases in kindergarten children during a routine school task, manuscript submitted to *Child Development*, 1984. See J. J. Lynch, *The Language of the Heart* for description. See also J. J. Lynch and W. H. Gantt, The heart rate component of the social reflex in dogs: The conditional effects of petting and person, *Conditional Reflex* 3:2 (1968):69–80. S. A. Thomas, et al., Changes in nurses' blood pressure and heart rate while communicating, *Journal of Research in Nursing and Health* 7 (1984):119–26.

168 Veterans Administration Cooperative Study Group on Antihypertensive Agents, Effects of treatment on morbidity in hypertension:

Results in patients with diastolic pressure averaging 115 through 129 mm Hg, *Journal of the American Medical Association* 202 (1967):1028–34. Veterans Administration Cooperative Study Group on Antihypertensive Agents, Effects of treatment on morbidity in hypertension: Results in patients with diastolic pressure averaging 90 through 114 mm Hg, *Journal of the American Medical Association* 213 (1970):1143–52.

170 Michael's case is described in Lynch's *The Language of the Heart*.

172 Lynch's technical studies, soon to be issued in a book, are quite important. See J. J. Lynch et al., The effects of human contact on the heart activity of curarized patients in a shock-trauma unit, *American Heart Journal* 88 (1974):160–69. J. J. Lynch et al., The effects of human contact on cardiac arrhythmia in coronary care patients, *Journal of Nervous and Mental Disease* 158 (1974):88–99. J. J. Lynch et al., Human contact and cardiac arrhythmia in a coronary care unit, *Psychosomatic Medicine* 39 (1977):188–92. S. A. Thomas, J. J. Lynch, and M. E. Mills, Psychosocial influences on heart arrhythmia in a coronary care patient, *Heart and Lung* 4 (1975):746–50. J. J. Lynch et al., Psychological aspects of cardiac arrhythmia, *American Heart Journal* 93 (1977):645–57. J. J. Lynch et al., Blood pressure changes while talking, *Israeli Journal of Medical Science* 18:5 (1982):575–79. Lynch's teacher has also had great influence: W. H. Gantt, The role of teleology in behavior, editorial, *Pavlovian Journal of Biological Science* 14:3 (1979):157–59.

Chapter 12: A Heart Apart

174 R. H. Rosenman, R. J. Brand, C. D. Jenkins, M. Friedman, et al., Coronary heart disease in the Western Collaborative Study: Final follow-up experience of eight and one-half years, *Journal of the American Medical Association* 223 (1975):872–77.

175 Drawn from the classic descriptions of Type A behavior. See M. Friedman and R. H. Rosenman, *Type A Behavior and Your Heart* (New York: Alfred A. Knopf, 1974).

178 The excerpts from interviews with Type A and B individuals were provided by Dr. Charles Swencionis.

179 M. Friedman and D. Ulmer, *Treating Type A Behavior and Your Heart* (New York: Alfred A. Knopf, 1984).

181 T. M. Dembrowski, J. M. MacDougall, R. S. Eliot, and J. C. Buell, Moving beyond Type A, *Advances* 1 (1984):16–26.

182 For a current and thorough review of the role of anger and hostility in cardiovascular disease see M. Chesney and R. H. Rosenman,

eds., *Anger and Hostility in Cardiovascular and Behavioral Disorders* (Washington: Hemisphere Publishing Corp., 1985).

184 For a thorough review of the evidence linking self-involvement and heart disease see L. Scherwitz, L. E. Graham, and D. Ornish, Self-involvement and the risk factors for coronary heart disease, *Advances* 2 (1985):6–18. Also L. Scherwitz, R. McKelvain, C. Laman, et al., Type A behavior, self-involvement, and coronary atherosclerosis, *Psychosomatic Medicine* 45 (1983):47–57.

186 G. L. Engel, Sudden and rapid death during psychological stress: Folklore or folk wisdom, *Annals of Internal Medicine* 74 (1971):771–82. In another study of 117 patients who underwent emergency resuscitation for life-threatening heart rhythm disturbances, 25 reported a serious interpersonal conflict in the twenty-four hours before the episode. In one instance, a Yankee fan went into ventricular fibrillation as he watched his team lose to the Red Sox. See B. Lown, R. A. DeSilva, P. Reich, and B. J. Murawski, Psychophysiologic factors in sudden cardiac death, *American Journal of Psychiatry* 137 (1980):1325–35.

187 For a recent review of sudden death and the work of Dr. James Skinner see D. Monagan, Sudden death, *Discover* 7:1 (1986):64–71. Also see B. Lown, R. L. Verrier, and S. H. Rabinowitz, Neural and psychologic mechanisms and the problem of sudden cardiac death, *The American Journal of Cardiology* 39 (1977):890–902.

Chapter 13: Friends Can Be Good Medicine

191 For an excellent discussion of the impact of the physical and social environment see R. Lindheim and S. L. Syme, Environments, people, and health, *Annual Review of Public Health* 4 (1983):335–59.

191 H. J. Gans, *The Urban Villagers: Group and Class in the Life of Italian-Americans* (New York: Free Press, 1962). M. Fried, Grieving for a lost home, in *The Urban Condition*, ed. L. Duhl (New York: Basic Books, 1963).

192 The weak social support given to cancer patients is described in G. W. Mitchell and A. S. Glicksman, Cancer patients: Knowledge and attitudes, *Cancer* 40 (1977):61–66. The nature of social support for widows is discussed in K. N. Walker, A. MacBride, and M. L. S. Vachon, Social support networks and the crisis of bereavement, *Social Science and Medicine* 11 (1977):35–41.

192 J. Medalie and V. Goldbourt, Angina pectoris among 10,000 men: II. Psychosocial and other risk factors as evidenced by a multivariate analysis of a five-year incidence study. *American Journal of Med-*

icine 60 (1976):910–21. J. Medalie, M. Snyder, J. J. Groen, H. N. Neufeld, V. Goldbourt, and E. Riss, Angina pectoris among 10,000 men: 5 year incidence and univariate analysis, *American Journal of Medicine* 55 (1973):583–94.

193 H. Morowitz, Hiding in the Hammond Report, *Hospital Practice* (August 1975):35–39.

193 The extract is from C. F. Longino and A. Lipman, Married and spouseless men and women in planned retirement communities: Support network differentials, *Journal of Marriage and the Family* 43 (1981):169–77.

194 For a study of the differential effects of divorce on mental health problems in men and women see N. Gerstel and C. Riesman, Social networks in a vulnerable population: The separated and divorced, paper presented at the American Public Health Association Meetings, Los Angeles, CA, November 4, 1981.

195 B. Raphael, Preventive intervention with the recently bereaved, *Archives of General Psychiatry* 34 (1977):1450–54. M. L. S. Vachon, W. A. L. Lyall, J. Rogers, K. Freedman-Letofsky, and S. J. J. Freeman, A controlled study of self-help intervention for widows, *American Journal of Psychiatry* 137 (1980):1380–84.

195 R. Sosa, J. Kennell, M. Klaus, S. Robertson, and J. Urrutia, The effect of a supportive companion on perinatal problems, length of labor, and mother-infant interaction, *New England Journal of Medicine* 303 (1980):597–600.

196 D. E. Morisky, N. M. DeMuth, M. Field-Fass, L. W. Green, and D. M. Levine, Evaluation of family health education to build social support for long-term control of high blood pressure, *Health Education Quarterly* 12 (1985):35–50. D. E. Morisky, D. M. Levine, L. W. Green, S. Shapiro, R. P. Russell, and C. R. Smith, Five-year blood pressure control and mortality following health education for hypertensive patients, *American Journal of Public Health* 73 (1983): 153–62.

197 E. C. Devine and T. D. Cook, A meta-analytic analysis of effects of psychoeducational interventions on length of postsurgical hospital stay, *Nursing Research* 32 (1983):267–74. Also see E. Mumford, H. J. Schlesinger, and G. V. Glass, The effects of psychological intervention on recovery from surgery and heart attacks: An analysis of the literature, *American Journal of Public Health* 72 (1982):141–51.

197 M. Minkler, S. Frantz, and R. Wechsler, Social support and social action organizing in a "gray ghetto": The Tenderloin experience,

Quarterly of Community Health Education 3 (1982–83):3–15. *Working Together for a Better Life*, prepared by the Tenderloin Tenants for Safer Streets (Tenderloin Senior Outreach Project, 495 Ellis Street, No. 460, San Francisco, CA 95102), 1983.

199 B. B. Arnetz, T. Theorell, L. Levi, A. Kallner, and P. Eneroth, An experimental study of social isolation of elderly people: Psychoendocrine and metabolic effects. *Psychosomatic Medicine* 45 (1983):395–406.

200 E. J. Langer and J. Rodin, The effects of choice and enhanced personal responsibility for the aged: A field experiment in an institutional setting, *Journal of Personality and Social Psychology* 34 (1976):191–98; and J. Rodin and E. J. Langer, Long-term effects of a control-relevant intervention with the institutionalized aged, *Journal of Personality and Social Psychology* 35 (1977):897–902.

200 Certain jobs linked to hypertension, *Medical World News* (February 24, 1986).

Chapter 14: Feeling Bored, Feeling Blitzed

208 T. H. Holmes and R. H. Rahe, The social readjustment rating scale, *Journal of Psychosomatic Research* 11 (1967):213–18. Also see B. Dohrenwend and B. Dohrenwend, eds., *Stressful Life Events: Their Nature and Effects* (New York: John Wiley, 1974).

211 A. D. Kanner, J. C. Coyne, C. Schaefer, and R. S. Lazarus, Comparison of two modes of stress measurement: Daily hassles and uplifts versus major life events, *Journal of Behavioral Medicine* 4 (1981):1–39. R. S. Lazarus, Little hassles can be hazardous to health, *Psychology Today* 15 (1981):58–62. Preliminary research failed to demonstrate a moderating or protective effect from daily uplifts. For a discussion see R. S. Lazarus, Puzzles in the study of daily hassles, *Journal of Behavioral Medicine* 7 (1984):375–89.

212 See H. Selye, *The Stress of Life* (New York: McGraw-Hill, 1956) for the classic statement of the concept of stress. This initial conceptualization has been modified based on subsequent research and has been dissected into the relevant components as scientific investigation and understanding have progressed.

215 M. M. Haith, *Rules That Babies Look By: The Organization of Newborn Visual Activity* (New York: Lawrence Erlbaum, 1980). R. L. Fantz, The origin of form perception, *Scientific American* 204 (1961):66–72.

217 M. Zuckerman, Perceptual isolation as a stress situation—a review, *Archives of General Psychiatry* 11 (1964):225–276. M. Zuckerman and

M. M. Haber, Need for stimulation as a source of stress response to perceptual isolation, *Journal of Abnormal Psychology* 70 (1965): 371–77.

218 R. J. Wurtman, Nutrients that modify the brain, *Scientific American* 246:4 (1982):50. R. J. Wurtman and J. J. Wurtman, eds., *Nutrition and the Brain,* multivolume (New York: Raven Press, 1977–85).

219 A. P. Krueger and D. S. Sobel, Air ions and health, *Ways of Health* ed. D. Sobel.

219 N. E. Rosenthal, D. A. Sack, et al., Seasonal affective disorder: A description of the syndrome and preliminary findings with light therapy, *Archives of General Psychiatry* 41 (1984):72–80.

221 R. S. Ulrich, View through a window may influence recovery from surgery, *Science* 224 (1984):420–21.

221 See R. Ornstein, *The Psychology of Consciousness* for a discussion.

223 M. Diamond, Age, sex and environmental influences, in *Biological Foundations of Cerebral Dominance,* ed. Geschwind and Galaburda.

223 H. B. Andervont, Influence of environment on mammary cancer in mice, *Journal of the National Cancer Institute* 4 (1944):579–81. H. B. Andervont, Spontaneous tumors in a subline of strain C3H mice, *Journal of the National Cancer Institute* 1 (1941):737–44. O. Muhlbock, Influence of environment on the incidence of mammary tumors in mice, *Acta Unio Internationalis Contra Cancrum* 7 (1950):351–53.

225 J. T. Nix, Study of the relationship of environmental factors to the type and frequency of cancer causing death in nuns, *Hospital Progress* 45 (1964):71–74.

226 This discussion of understimulation, boredom, and cancer draws from Augustin M. de la Peña, *The Psychobiology of Cancer* (New York: Praeger Publishers, 1983) and a series of audiocassettes by de la Peña, "Boredom, understimulation and cancer" (ISHK Tapes, Box 1062, Cambridge, MA 02239, 1984). Also see the following: G. Newton, C. G. Bly, and C. McCrary, Effects of early experience on the response to transplanted tumors, *Journal of Nervous and Mental Disorders* 134 (1962):522–27. J. Achterberg, G. F. Lawlis, O. C. Simon, and S. Simonton, Psychological factors and blood chemistries as disease outcome predictors for cancer patients, *Multivariate Clinical and Experimental Research* 3 (1977):107–22. J. Achterberg, I. Collerrain, and P. Craig, A possible relationship between cancer, mental retardation and mental disorder, *Social Science and Medicine*

12 (1978):135–39. V. N. Fadeeva, *Pavlov Journal of Higher Nervous Activity* 1 (1951):165.

227 R. Karasek, D. Baker, F. Marxer, A. Ahlbom, and T. Theorell, Job decision latitude, job demands, and cardiovascular disease: A prospective study of Swedish men, *American Journal of Public Health* 71 (1981):694–705. L. Alfredson, R. Karasek, and T. Theorell, Myocardial infarction risk and psychological work environment: An analysis of the male Swedish working force, *Social Science and Medicine* 16 (1982):463–73.

Chapter 15: Of Hardiness, Coherence, and Stability

230 E. E. Werner and R. S. Smith, *Vulnerable, But Invincible: A Study of Resilient Children* (New York: McGraw-Hill, 1982). For additional studies of stress resistance in children see N. Garmezy and M. Rutter, eds., *Stress, Coping and Development in Children* (New York: McGraw-Hill, 1983). N. Garmezy and A. Tellegen, Studies of stress-resistant children: Methods, variables, and preliminary findings, in *Applied Developmental Psychology,* ed. F. J. Morrison, C. Lord, and D. Keating (Orlando: Academic Press, 1984).

233 S. R. Maddi and S. C. Kobasa, *The Hardy Executive: Health Under Stress* (Homewood, IL: Dow Jones-Irwin, 1984). S. O. Kobasa, How much stress can you survive? *American Health* 3 (September 1984):64–77. S. C. Kobasa, Stressful life events, personality and health: An inquiry into hardiness, *Journal of Personality and Social Psychology* 37 (1979):1–11. M. Pines, Psychological hardiness: The role of challenge in health, *Psychology Today* (December 1980): 34–44.

237 S. C. Kobasa, S. Maddi, and S. Kahn, Hardiness and health: A prospective study, *Journal of Personality and Social Psychology* 42 (1982):168–77.

238 S. C. Kobasa, S. R. Maddi, and S. Courington, Personality and constitution as mediators in the stress-illness relationship. *Journal of Health and Social Behavior* 22 (1981):368–78. S. C. Kobasa, S. R. Maddi, and M. C. Puccetti, Personality and exercise as buffers in the stress-illness relationship, *Journal of Behavioral Medicine* 4 (1982):391–404. S. C. Kobasa and M. C. Puccetti, Personality and social resources in stress-resistance, *Journal of Personality and Social Psychology* 45 (1983):839–50.

239 For an in-depth exploration of the costs and benefits of illusions and denial see S. Bresnitz, ed., *The Denial of Stress* (New York:

International Universities Press, 1983); and D. Goleman, Denial and hope, *American Health* 3 (December 1984):54–61.

240 R. Lazarus, Positive denial: The case for not facing reality, *Psychology Today* (November 1979):44–60.

240 D. Goleman, *Vital Lies, Simple Truths: The Psychology of Self-Deception* (New York: Simon and Schuster, 1985).

241 H. Staudenmayer, R. A. Kinsman, J. F. Dirks, S. L. Spector, and C. Wangaard, Medical outcome in asthmatic patients: Effects of airways hyperreactivity and symptom-focused anxiety, *Psychosomatic Medicine* 41 (1979):109–18.

241 F. Cohen, R. S. Lazarus, Active coping processes, coping dispositions, and recovery from surgery, *Psychosomatic Medicine* 35 (1973):375–89.

242 R. Lazarus, Positive denial: The case for not facing reality, *Psychology Today* (November 1979): 44–60.

242 T. P. Hackett, N. H. Cassem, and H. A. Wishnie, The coronary care unit: An appraisal of its psychological hazards, *New England Journal of Medicine* 279 (1968):1365–70. T. P. Hackett and N. H. Cassem, Psychological management of the myocardial infarction patient, *Journal of Human Stress* 1 (1975):25–38.

244 M. Seligman, *Learned Helplessness* (San Francisco: W. H. Freeman & Co, 1975).

245 For a review of role of hope in therapeutic relationships see J. G. Bruhn, Therapeutic value of hope, *Southern Medical Journal* 77 (1984):215–19.

245 A. Schmale and H. Iker, The effect of hopelessness and the development of cancer: I. Identification of uterine cervical cancer in women with atypical cytology, *Psychosomatic Medicine* 28 (1966): 714–21. A. Schmale and H. Iker, Hopelessness as a predictor of cervical cancer, *Social Science and Medicine* 5 (1971):95–100.

245 D. Spence, The paradox of denial, *The Denial of Stress*, ed. S. Bresnitz.

246 R. C. Mason, G. Clark, R. B. Reeves, and B. Wagner, Acceptance and healing, *Journal of Religion and Health* 8 (1969):123–30.

246 Shlomo Bresnitz interview by Daniel Goleman: To dream the impossible dream, *American Health* 3 (December 1984):60–61.

247 K. Gravelle, Can a feeling of capability reduce arthritis pain? *Advances* 2 (1985):8–13. K. Lorig, J. Laurin, and H. Holman, Arthritis

self-management: A study of the effectiveness of patient education for the elderly, *The Gerontologist* 24 (1984):455–57. S. Lenker, K. Lorig, and D. Gallagher, Reasons for the lack of association between changes in health behavior and improved health status: An exploratory study, *Patient Education and Counseling* 6 (1984): 69–72.

248 For a discussion of the self-efficacy theory developed by Albert Bandura, see A. Bandura, Self-efficacy mechanism in human agency, *American Psychologist* 37 (1982):122–47. For a review of perceived self-efficacy applied to smoking cessation relapse, pain experience and management, control of eating and weight, success of recovery from myocardial infarction, and adherence to preventive health programs, see A. O'Leary, Self-efficacy and health, *Behavioral Research and Therapy* 23 (1985):437–51.

249 A. Bandura, C. B. Taylor, S. L. Williams, I. N. Mefford, and J. D. Barchas, Catecholamine secretion as a function of perceived self-efficacy, *Journal of Consulting and Clinical Psychology* 53 (1985): 406–14.

249 The findings of the Manitoba Longitudinal Study on Aging are reported in J. M. Mossey and E. Shapiro, Self-rated health: A predictor of mortality among the elderly, *American Journal of Public Health* 72 (1982):800–807.

250 The findings of the study of Alameda County residents are reported in G. A. Kaplan and T. Camacho, Perceived health and mortality: A nine-year follow-up of the Human Population Laboratory cohort, *American Journal of Epidemiology* 117 (1983):292–304.

251 A. Antonovsky, *Health, Stress, and Coping* (San Francisco: Jossey-Bass, 1979). For a later formulation of his concept of sense of coherence see A. Antonovsky, The sense of coherence as a determinant of health, in *Behavioral Health*, ed. J. D. Matarazzo, S. M. Weiss, J. A. Herd, N. E. Miller, and S. M. Weiss (New York: John Wiley, 1984); and A. Antonovsky, *Unravelling the Mystery of Health: How People Manage Stress and Stay Well* (San Francisco: Jossey-Bass, 1987).

252 Antonovosky in the chapter cited above (p. 120) makes the case even stronger for distinguishing health from other desirable social values:

> Those of us who study health, which we value, confront a strong temptation. It would be deeply satisfying if the characteristics that we personally value and find pleasing were also good for health. It is not at all accidental that a theme runs through the literature that mature, autono-

mous, creative, warm, and so on, people are also healthy. I would urgently warn against such a misinterpretation of the sense of coherence. To put it bluntly, a person with a strong sense of coherence might well be a terrible person in terms of my (or your) values. Such a person might well be a Nazi or, to bring it closer to home, a highly manipulative, unscrupulous academic, or a member of an extreme religious sect. True believers—keeping in mind the warning about the fake sense of coherence—are likely to have a strong sense of coherence.

256 R. S. Eliot and D. L. Breo, *Is It Worth Dying For?* (New York: Bantam, 1984).

257 Shah's statement is found in *An Advanced Understanding of Man,* audiocassette tape (ISHK, Cambridge, MA, 1984).

FOR FURTHER READING

Advances: Journal of the Institute for the Advancement of Health (Institute for the Advancement of Health, 16 East 53d Street, New York, NY 10022). This professional quarterly journal, initiated in 1983, examines important developments in the emerging interdisciplinary investigation of how mind-body interactions affect health and disease. It is a virtual gold mine of articles, reviews, and abstracts exploring the connections between the central nervous system and the immune system, the influence of feelings and behavior patterns on health, and the creation of new medical treatments which include mental and behavioral interventions.

Antonovsky, Aaron. *Health, Stress, and Coping.* San Francisco: Jossey-Bass, 1979. This is a seminal work by a medical sociologist who explores the question of how it is that anyone is healthy given all the inevitable stressors of life. He considers the commonalities behind the resources which help people resist stress and introduces the central theoretical construct of sense of coherence. For an updated discussion of sense of coherence see also A. Antonovosky, The sense of coherence as a determinant of health, in J. D. Matarazzo, S. M. Weiss, J. A. Herd, N. E. Miller, and S. M. Weiss, eds. *Behavioral Health.* New York: John Wiley, 1984; and A. Antonovsky, *Unravelling the Mystery of Health: How People Manage Stress and Stay Well.* San Francisco: Jossey-Bass, 1987.

Benson, Herbert. *The Relaxation Response*. New York: William Morrow, 1975.
——. *The Mind/Body Effect*. New York: Simon & Schuster, 1979.
——. *Beyond the Relaxation Response*. New York: Times Books, 1984.
A trio of highly popular books by the Harvard cardiologist who has investigated the health effects of relaxation and meditation.
Cohen, Sheldon, and S. Leonard Syme, eds. *Social Support and Health*. New York: Academic Press, 1985.
This collection of seventeen articles is the best current single-volume discussion of the promise and pitfalls in the research linking social support and health. The articles are somewhat technical as the authors explore the definitions of social support, research methods, and the findings on the importance of social support in children, the middle-aged, and the elderly.
Dubos, René. *Mirage of Health*. New York: Doubleday & Co., 1959.
——. *Man Adapting*. New Haven: Yale University Press, 1965.
Dubos has written perhaps more clearly and with greater insight than anyone else on health and disease as expressions of human adaptation to changing environments. A microbiologist by training, he was one of the first to recognize the importance of ecological rather than medical factors in the decline of infectious diseases. A pleasure to read.
Eliot, Robert, and Dennis Breo. *Is It Worth Dying for?* New York: Bantam, 1984.
Perhaps the most readable of all the "save your heart" books. It gives a good overview on the evidence about "hot reactors."
Cousins, Norman. *Anatomy of an Illness*. New York: Bantam, 1981.
——. *The Healing Heart*. New York: W. W. Norton, 1983.
Two highly readable, personal accounts of Cousins's encounters with two life-threatening illnesses, one a serious arthritic condition and the other a heart attack. He argues that the power of positive moods, thoughts, and attitudes plays a vital role in the recovery from illness.
Frank, Jerome. *Persuasion and Healing*. Baltimore: Johns Hopkins Press, 1973.
In this highly readable book, Frank investigates such diverse therapeutic approaches as shamanism, faith healing, religious revivalism, the placebo effect, and the modern psychotherapies. He finds some striking commonalities, including the ability of the healer to mobilize expectant faith, restore morale, and alter the beliefs of the patient.
Gentry, Doyle W., ed. *Handbook of Behavioral Medicine*. New York: The Guilford Press, 1984.
This is an outstanding collection of review articles covering the role of behavioral, psychosocial, and cultural factors in health and disease. It includes articles on behavior and the immune, gastrointestinal, and cardiovascular systems as well as discussions of stress, coping, and

community-based interventions to decrease risk of cardiovascular disease. It is written primarily for a professional audience.

Locke, Steven, and Douglas Colligan. *The Healer Within.* New York: E. P. Dutton, 1986.

An exciting account of the historic roots and modern emergence of the field of psychoneuroimmunology—the scientific study of the mind, the nervous system, and the immune system. Written in a lively style for a general readership, it explores how stress (and hope) may affect immune function and, thereby, influence susceptibility to a wide variety of diseases.

Lynch, James. *The Broken Heart.* New York: Basic Books, 1977.

——. *The Language of the Heart,* Basic Books, 1985.

In our opinion perhaps the most seminal contribution on how the mind, the heart, and the social world are related. Lynch's work is at that point where what seems obvious to many people suddenly leaps into a scientific breakthrough. Cardiologists reading Lynch have been known to say, "Of course that's all true," while going about their work ignoring the implications of how they may well be influencing the heart functions of their patients, and how social conditions may lie at the root of many of the disorders.

McKeown, Thomas. *The Role of Medicine: Dream, Mirage or Nemesis?* Princeton, NJ: Princeton University Press, 1979.

This book provides the best, most readable summary of the debate on the determinants of health. McKeown analyzes the available data and argues that the major improvements in health were due more to environmental and behavioral changes rather than medical care. He also maintains that future improvements in health lie more in an understanding of the environmental and behavioral origins of disease and subsequent prevention than in specific medical treatments.

Matarazzo, Joseph D., Sharlene M. Weiss, J. Alan Herd, Neal E. Miller, and Stephen M. Weiss, eds. *Behavioral Health.* New York: John Wiley, 1984.

This mammoth 1,290-page volume brings together the most comprehensive collection of articles on the role of behavior in determining health. Though aimed primarily at an interdisciplinary professional audience, most of the articles are appropriate for a general reader. It covers the standard areas of exercise, diet, smoking, blood pressure, safety, and drug abuse. Additionally, it contains some fascinating articles on sense of coherence, self-efficacy, placebos, compliance, coping with stress, and psychoimmunology.

Pelletier, Kenneth R. *Mind as Healer, Mind as Slayer.* New York: Delta, 1977.

——. *Holistic Medicine: From Stress to Optimal Health.* New York: Delta, 1979.

Two early books that review the research linking psychosocial stress

and various diseases as well as a discussion of methods of stress
management such as relaxation and biofeedback training.

Ornstein, Robert. *The Psychology of Consciousness*. New York: Viking-
Penguin, 1986.
An expanded discussion of how the nervous system calculates a rep-
resentation of the world.

Ornstein, Robert, Richard Thompson, and David Macaulay. *The Amazing Brain*. Boston: Houghton Mifflin, 1984.
A visual and intellectual exploration into the history, evolution, con-
struction, and chemical and electrical operation of the only object we
know of that is able to contemplate, study, and describe itself. This
step-by-step discussion of the brain is illuminated with amazing
drawings.

Sobel, David S., ed. *Ways of Health: Holistic Approaches in Ancient and
Contemporary Medicine*. New York: Harcourt Brace Jovanovich, 1979.
A collection of twenty essays discussing the limitations of modern
medicine, various ancient and unorthodox systems of healing such as
Navaho and Chinese medicine, forms of self-regulation such as yoga
and biofeedback, and the ramifications of a changing environment on
health. The essays argue for an integration of the technical achievements of Western scientific medicine with the psychosocial speciali-
zations of ancient and unorthodox medicine.

White, Leonard, Bernard Tursky, and Gary E. Schwartz, eds. *Placebo:
Theory, Research and Mechanisms*. New York: The Guilford Press, 1985.
This collection of twenty-five technical articles covers all aspects of
placebos: from theory, philosophy, and ethics to clinical phenomena
and the use of placebos in research. Several authors present intriguing explanations of how placebos work.

INDEX

acetylcholine, 65, 88, 218
Achterberg, Jeanne, 225
acne, 79
ACTH (adrenocorticotrophic
    hormone), 44, 94, 178–79, 212
action-emotion complex, 175
acupuncture, 95
addiction, 93
Ader, Robert, 141–42
ADH (antidiuretic hormone), 48
adipose tissue, 50
adrenal glands, 65, 94, 212
adrenaline, 180, 185; see also
    catecholamines; epinephrine
aggressiveness:
    life expectancy and, 68
    in Type A Behavior Pattern, 175,
        179
AIDS (acquired immune deficiency
    syndrome), 145–46
Akil, Huda, 94
Alameda County, Calif., population
    study, 122–23, 250
alcohol, health and, 26
alienation, 156, 157, 235
Allen, Woody, 136
allergies, 24
    hypnosis as treatment for, 102–3
    immune system and, 103, 143, 145,
        146, 150, 151
Amazing Brain, The (Ornstein,
    Thompson, and Macaulay), 36
ambition, 176, 185
amino acids, 92
amphetamine, 225
analgesics, 93, 95, 98
anaphylactic shock, 146
Anderson, John, 119
Andervont, H. B., 223
Andres, Reuben, 52
anemia, 82, 147
    acquired hemolytic, 146
    pernicious, 146
anesthesia, hypnotic, 99
anger, see emotions; hostility
angina pectoris, 79, 181

antagonists, 91
anthrax, 28
antibiotics, 19, 21, 24
    streptomycin, 18, 22, 43
antibodies, 141, 152, 155, 156
antidepressants, 188
antigens, 143, 144, 146, 150
antisepsis, 30
antitoxin, 24
Antonovsky, Aaron, 250–51
anxiety:
    adrenaline and, 185
    cancer and, 156
    childbirth and, 196
    endorphins and, 93
    fear vs., 66–67
    placebo effect and, 79, 83
    separation and, 134
appendicitis, 24
ARC (AIDS-related complex), 146
Aristotle, 43
Arnetz, Bengt, 199
arthritis, 24, 30
    coping with, 247–48
    genetic factors in, 147
    placebo effect on, 79
    rheumatoid, 146, 147–48, 151
    social and psychological factors in,
        119, 147, 247–48
aspirin, 44, 86–87
asthma, 24, 119, 151, 241
    crying and, 44
    placebo effect on, 79
atherosclerosis, 127
attachment (bonding), 134–35, 156,
    231
autoimmune diseases, 143, 145, 146–
    148, 151
"avoidance coping," 236

Bandura, Albert, 249
Barthrop, R. W., 138
B-cells, 144
Beecher, Henry, 79, 82–83
Berkman, Lisa, 122

symptoms (*cont.*)
    of SLE, 146–47
    sneezing, 45
    of "sweating sickness," 20
    thirst, 48
    vomiting, 79, 84–85
    weight loss, 82
syphilis, 19, 24, 29

tachistoscope, 61
"target cells," 38
taste, 45, 62
T-cells, 139, 144, 145, 149, 150, 152,
    153
tears, composition of, 44
Tecumseh, Mich., death rate in, 123
temperature, body:
    brain's control of, 38, 41, 43, 47,
        149
    high (fever), 17, 44, 146, 147
    hypnosis and, 98
    low, 135
temporal lobes, 57
Tenderloin Senior Outreach Project
    197–99
Teresa of Calcutta, Mother (Agnes
    Gonxha Bojaxhiu), 159–160,
    185
"terrain," 28–29
testosterone, 149, 199
tetanus, 24
thirst, 47–48
"thirst substance," 48
Thompson, Dick, 36
thymus, 140, 144, 148, 150
thyroid disorders, 149
thyroid hormone, 148
time urgency, 175, 177, 182, 185
tobacco:
    health and, 26, 193
    heart disease and, 31, 178
toxins, 145
Transactional Psychophysiology,
    171
triglycerides, 178
Trosseau, Armand, 83–84
tuberculosis, 17, 18, 21–23, 29, 30,
    119, 145
    deaths from (chart), 22
tumors, 19, 101, 144, 151, 152, 157,
    158, 225
    benign vs. malignant, 223
    see also cancer

Type A Behavior Pattern 173–84, 188
    naming of, 179
Type B Behavior Pattern, 175, 176,
    177–78, 180
typhoid fever, 20

ulcers, 79
Ulmer, Diane, 179, 181
Ulrich, Roger, 220
urine, thirst and, 48
Utah, death rate in, 25–26
uterine cancer, 18, 82

Vachon, M. L. S., 195
Van Slyke, C. J., 179
varicose veins, 132
vasodepressor syncope, 188–89
vasodilation, 47
ventricular fibrillation, 186–88
ventricular tachycardia, 162
viruses, 24, 144
    Epstein-Barr, 152
    herpes simplex, 145, 152–53, 155
    HTLV-III, 146
    interferon and, 143
    polio, 23
    replication of, 143
    respiratory, 20
    in warts, 101
vision:
    blurred, 168
    brain's interpretation of, 107–8
    of newborns, 215
    stereoscopic, 63
    stimulation of, 215–16
    see also eyes
visualization and guided imagery,
    153–55
vomiting:
    chemotherapy and, 84–85
    placebos and, 79
Vulnerable, but Invincible (Werner and
    Smith), 230

Warsaw Ghetto, 51
warts, 99–102
    folk remedies for, 100–101
    hypnosis as cure for, 99–100, 101
    spontaneous regression of, 101
Wayne, John, 163
WCGS (Western Collaborative Group
    Study), 178, 181
weather-sensitive people, 218–19